American Tang Soo Do Hyungs

A Guide to Black Belt

By Courtney A. Griner

American Tang Soo Do Hyungs
A Guide to Black Belt

Disclaimer

It is important to understand that the authors and publisher of this instructional book cannot be held responsible for any injuries that may occur while attempting the techniques or following the instructions provided. Martial arts training can be hazardous, both to yourself and to others, if not practiced safely. It is recommended that you seek guidance from a qualified martial arts instructor before attempting any of the techniques outlined in this book. Additionally, as the physical demands of these activities may be too intense for certain individuals, it is imperative that you consult with a physician prior to beginning training.

Published by Patmos Publishing LLC, 2023

ISBN: 979-8-9867371-4-0 (Paperback)

For information contact:
Patmos Publishing LLC
www.patmospublishing.com

Table of Contents

Author 1

History 2

How To Tie Your Belt 5

Kicho Hyung 7

Kicho Hyung Il Bu 8

Kicho Hyung Ee Bu 11

Kicho Hyung Sahm Bu 14

Pyung Ahn Hyung 18

Pyung Ahn Cho Dan 19

Pyung Ahn Ee Dan 23

Pyung Ahn Sahm Dan 27

Pyung Ahn Sah Dan 31

Pyung Ahn Oh Dan 35

Bassai Hyung 39

Bassai 40

Resource 46

Author

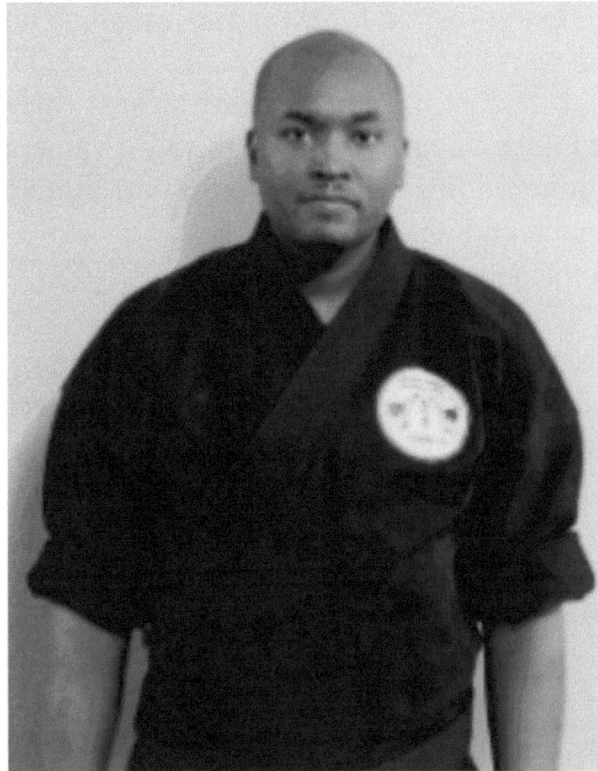

Courtney A. Griner
Practicing Martial Arts Since 1990

Ranks Earned:
American Tang Soo Do: 4th Degree Black Belt
IKCA Chinese Kenpo: 4th Degree Black Belt
BKF Karate: 4th Degree Black Belt

Active member of the Black Karate Federation (B.K.F.)
The Black Karate Federation, which was founded in late 1969, emerged on the Southern California Karate Tournament Circuit with a mission to level the playing field for black fighters, who were often cheated out of their victories and overlooked on the tournament circuits of the 1960s and 1970s. The BKF passionately believed in the power of martial arts to shape and transform young lives, offering after-school programs for children, affordable karate lessons for disadvantaged youth, and support and assistance for at-risk teens. Today, the BKF has expanded its reach across the world, continuing to inspire and empower young people of all ethnicities through the martial arts. ***See page 46.***

History

Koreans have lived in the same area for thousands of years and have a long history of trade, conflict, and warfare, both inside their own country and with adjacent countries and peoples. Interactions between the various tribes that inhabit modern-day China, Japan, and Okinawa have exposed the Korean people to a wide range of martial arts styles. Although it is impossible to establish an accurate timeline in the development of the ancient Korean martial arts, we can examine some of the significant events that influenced their growth.

Three Empires: The Korean peninsula was divided into three kingdoms two thousand years ago: Silla was established in 57 BC, Goguryeo in 37 BC, and Baekje in 18 BC. Together, Silla in the east and Baekje in the west controlled roughly the southern two-thirds of what is now South Korea. Goguryeo was much larger and encompassed the entirety of North Korea, a portion of Chinese Manchuria, and the northern third of South Korea today. In 668 AD, the Silla Dynasty brought the three kingdoms together after a long series of wars. Studying martial arts was very popular during this conflict, as evidenced by the numerous mural paintings and ruins that still exist that depict ancient martial arts. The "Hwarang," a group of young aristocratic warriors in Silla, combined and refined earlier forms of martial arts to create a new, more formal style. These warriors were the commanders and leaders during the contentions that brought about the unification of the Korean Peninsula under the new Silla Dynasty (668 AD–935 AD). The spiritual and technical roots of the majority of Korean martial arts can be found in this group. In fact, this heritage is still reflected in the names of some contemporary Korean martial arts, such as Hwa Rang Do and Hwa Soo Do.

Development in the Middle Ages: A warlord by the name of Wang Geon overthrew the Silla Kingdom in 918 AD and established the new kingdom: Goryeo ruled for 474 years, from 918 to 1392 AD, before being overthrown by the Joseon Dynasty, which ruled for 500 years. Under the names Gwonbeop, Taekkyon, Soo Bahk, Tang Soo, and others, the forerunners of what is now known as Tang Soo Do became increasingly popular during the nearly 1,000-year period of the Goryeo Kingdom and the Joseon Dynasty. The oldest known book on Korean martial arts was written in 1790, known as the Muyedobotongji. This book provides evidence that a martial art known as "Subak" was practiced at the time.

The Modern Era: Korea came under increasing Japanese and western (European and American) influence in the middle to late 1800s. International recognition of Japanese sovereignty over Korea, administered by the Japanese military, began in 1910 and lasted until the Japanese surrendered in 1945, when World War II came to an end. Traditional Korean martial arts were outlawed and punishable by death during this time period, making it illegal to practice or teach them in Korea. While only a few Japanese martial arts, such as Judo, Kendo, and others, were permitted, ancient Korean martial arts like Taekkyeon were secretly practiced. The Korean Peninsula was divided into two occupation zones in 1945 following World War II. The Soviet Union occupied the northern half and established a communist state: the Republic of Korea (South Korea) was established in the southern part of the peninsula occupied by the United States following the Japanese surrender, while the Democratic People's Republic of Korea (North Korea) was established elsewhere. In South Korea, traditional Korean martial arts were no longer prohibited, and a number of training schools were soon established.

The Chung Do Kwan, founded by Won Kuk Lee, was the first of many martial arts schools to open across Korea after the Japanese occupation ended. Lee is credited with being the first person to use the term "Tang Soo Do" to describe the Korean fighting art that had evolved from a variety of other styles. "The Way of the Chinese Hand" was originally pronounced "Tang Soo Do" or "Dang Soo Do" in Korean. Most Americans now translate it as "The Way of the Open Hand".

Some of the people who contributed to the development of Taekwondo, Tang Soo Do, and Kong Soo Do are:

Hwang Kee, founder of the "Moo Duk Kwan"
Kyung Suk Lee, founder of the "Yun Mu Kwan"
Yoon Byung-in, founder of the "YMCA Kwon Bup Bu"
Won Kuk Lee, founder of the "Chung Do Kwan"
Byung Jik Ro, founder of the "Song Moo Kwan"

In 1959, the name "Taekwondo" was adopted after the other kwans agreed to merge. Hwang Kee's Moo Duk Kwan school, on the other hand, chose not to merge with the other kwans; thus, the name Tang Soo Do is still used today.

Today, despite the existence of numerous organizations, Tang Soo Do still continues to thrive. It is not regulated by a large umbrella organization. As a result, each martial arts school or organization uses its own curriculum and establishes its own set of standards.

The Styles That Contributed to Tang Soo Do

The majority of Tang Soo Do practitioners can trace their lineage to Grandmaster Hwang Kee. He was the founder of the martial arts dojang known as the Moo Duk Kwan ("School of Martial Virtue"). Throughout his life, Hwang Kee studied various martial arts styles, such as the Korean art of Taekkyon, Okinawan karate, Japanese Shotokan, and Chinese martial arts styles like Tai Chi and Gung Fu. It is from these styles that Moo Duk Kwan Tang Soo Do was founded. He would later abandon the name "Tang Soo Do" and begin referring to his art as "Soo Bahk Do."

Won Kuk Lee was another talented martial artist who also helped to shape the art of Tang Soo Do. He infused a lot of Shotokan into his teachings. He was the founder of the Chung Do Kwan ("School of the Blue Wave"). He would later abandon the name "Tang Soo Do" and begin referring to his art as "Taekwondo."

Tang Soo Do Training

Tang Soo Do training consists of forms or Hyungs, one-step sparring, free sparring, line work (executing kicks, punches, and blocks in a line), and self-defense techniques against kicks, punches, grabs, and various weapon attacks.

Tang Soo Do is the Korean version of Japanese Shotokan Karate.

How To Tie Your Belt

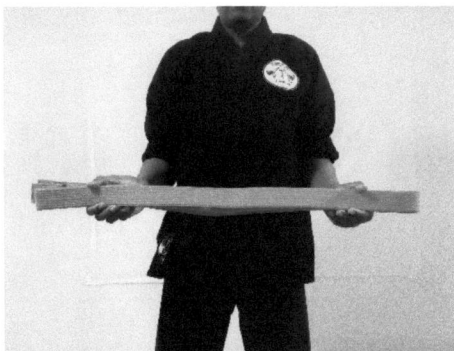

Start: Hold your belt in both hands.

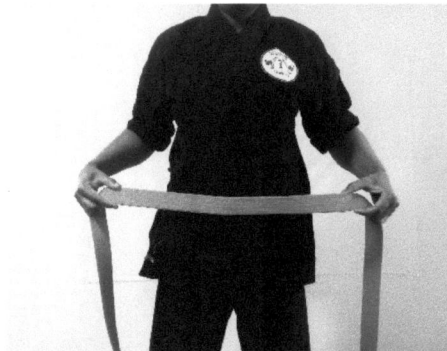

1. Place the middle section of your belt below your navel after unrolling it.

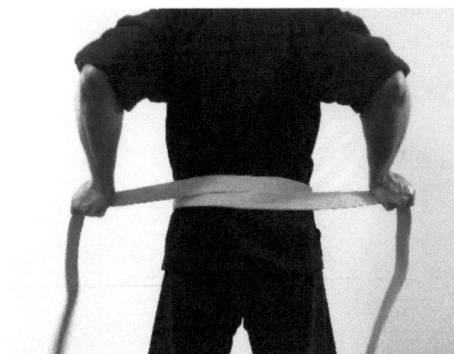

2. As shown, wrap the belt around your waist and cross over at the back.

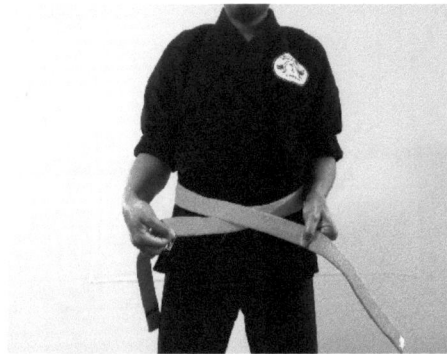

3. Cross over the top of the left-hand end by bringing the right side end around.

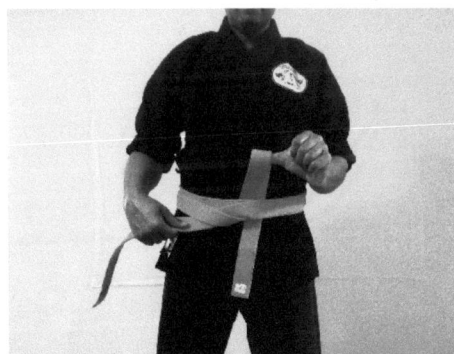

4. Between the uniform and the belt layers, pull the end of the right hand belt under and up.

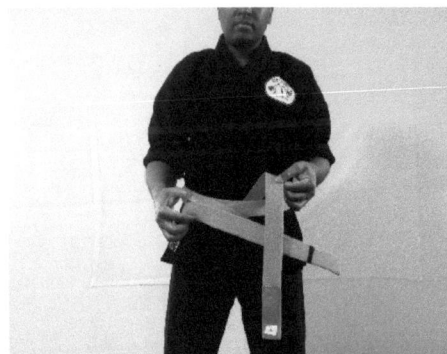

5. Pass through the loop and tie a knot by crossing the left-hand end over the right-hand end.

_**A**_

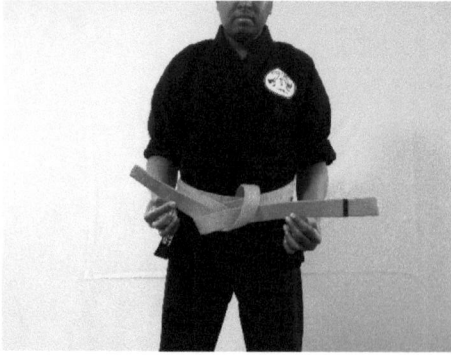

_B_

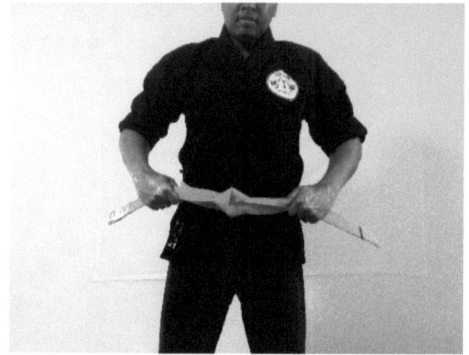

6. Pull your belt tightly at both ends.

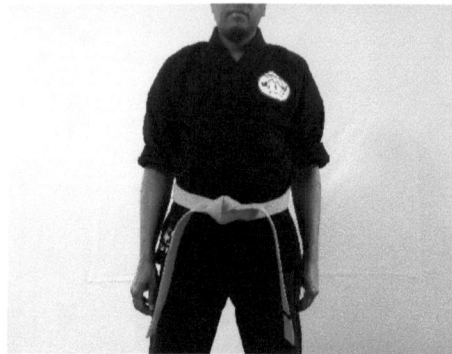

Finish

Kicho Hyung

White Belt

Orange Belt

Orange Belt I Stripe ▮

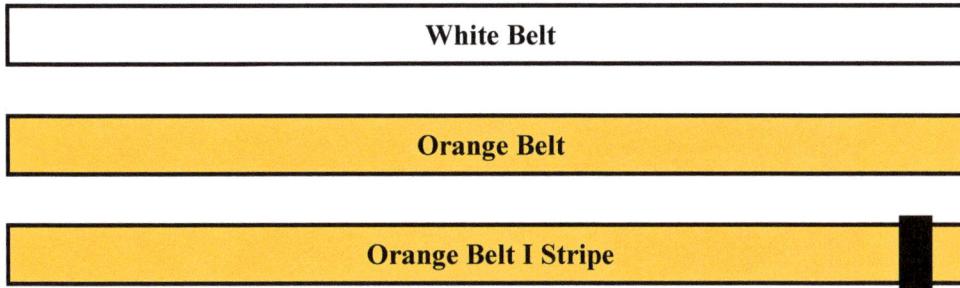

These three basic Hyungs have their roots in Japanese karate. In Shotokan these katas are known as: Taikyoku Shodan, Taikyoku Nidan, and Taikyoku Sandan. The initial Hyung, Kicho Hyung Il Bu, has not changed and is the same as Taikyoku Shodan. However, Kicho Hyung Ee Bu and Kicho Hyung Sahm Bu have experienced some slight changes.

1. Kicho Hyung Il Bu (Basic Form 1)

2. Kicho Hyung Ee Bu (Basic Form 2)

3. Kicho Hyung Sahm Bu (Basic Form 3)

Kicho Hyung Il Bu

Kicho Hyung Directions

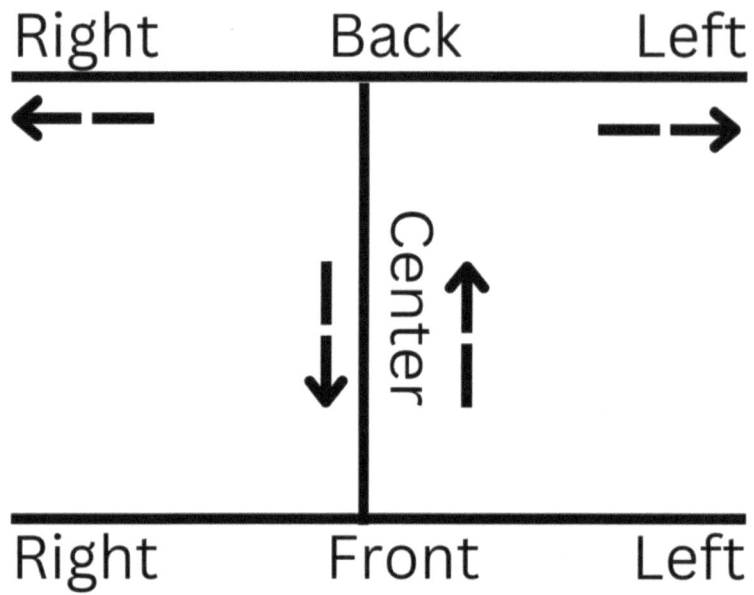

Right	Back	Left

← – –   – – →

↓ Center ↑

Right	Front	Left

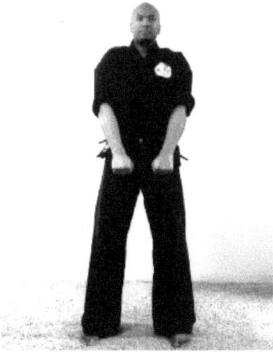

Start: Ready Stance
(Junbi Jase)

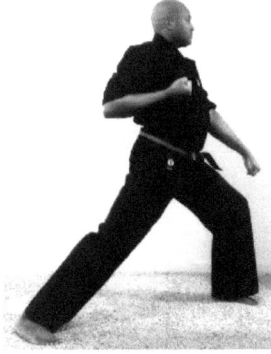

1. Turn Left 90 Degrees
Front Stance
Low Block

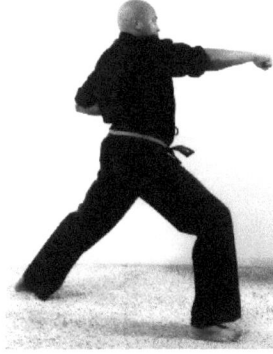

2. Step Forward
Front Stance
Middle Punch

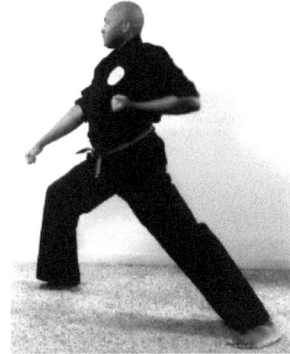

3. Turn Right 180 Degrees
Front Stance
Low Block

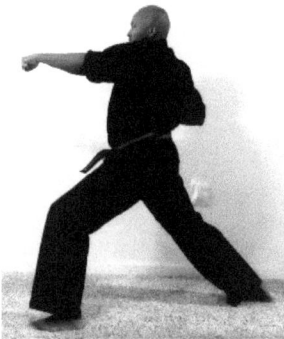

4. Step Forward
Front Stance
Middle Punch

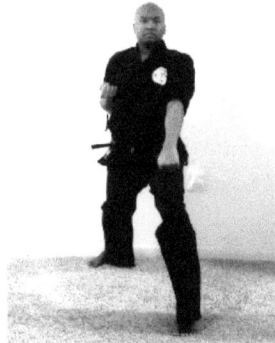

5. Turn Left 90 Degrees
Front Stance
Low Block

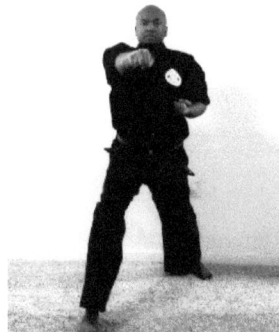

6. Step Forward
Front Stance
Middle Punch

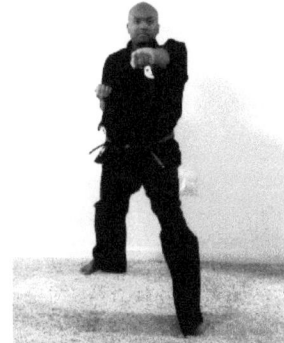

7. Step Forward
Front Stance
Middle Punch

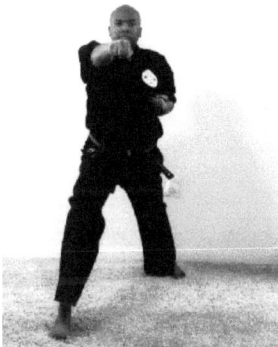

8. Step Forward
Front Stance
Middle Punch
Kihap!

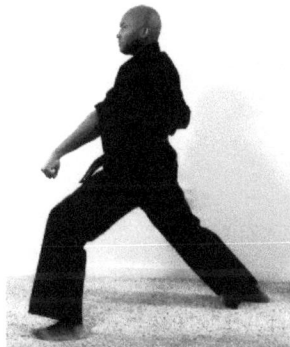

9. Turn Left 270 Degrees
Front Stance
Low Block

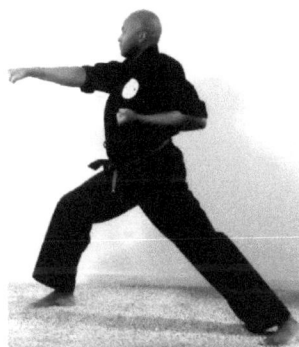

10. Step Forward
Front Stance
Middle Punch

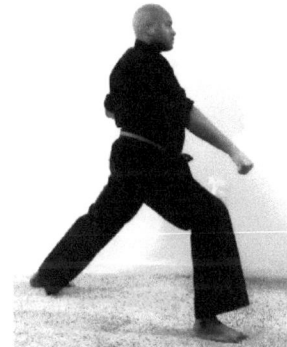

11. Turn Right 180 Degrees
Front Stance
Low Block

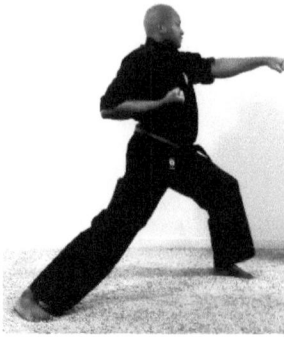

12. Step Forward
Front Stance
Middle Punch

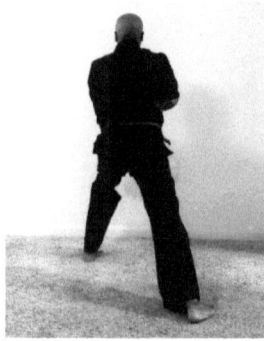

13. Turn Left 90 Degrees
Front Stance
Low Block

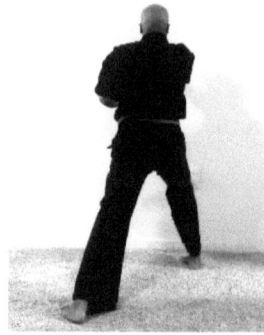

14. Step Forward
Front Stance
Middle Punch

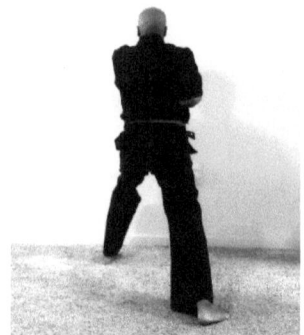

15. Step Forward
Front Stance
Middle Punch

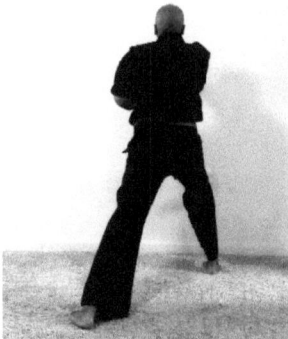

16. Step Forward
Front Stance
Middle Punch
Kihap!

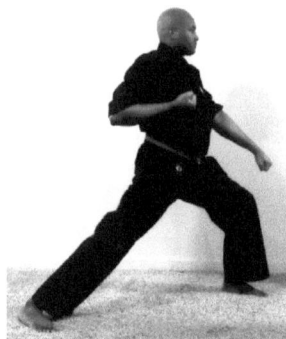

17. Turn Left 270 Degrees
Front Stance
Low Block

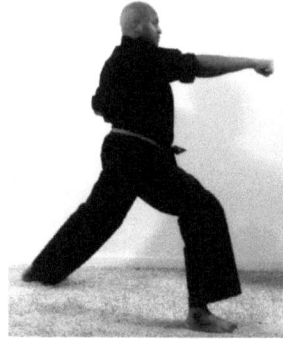

18. Step Forward
Front Stance
Middle Punch

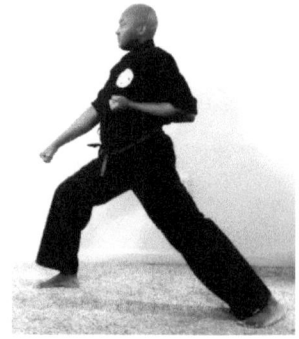

19. Turn Right 180 Degrees
Front Stance
Low Block

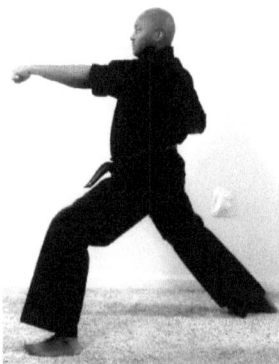

20. Step Forward
Front Stance
Middle Punch

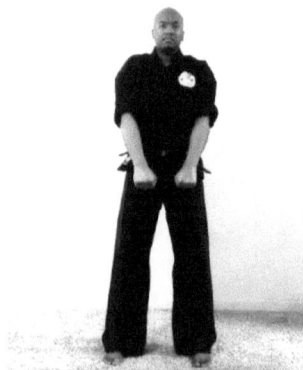

Finish: Ready Stance
(Junbi Jase)

Kicho Hyung Ee Bu

Kicho Hyung Directions

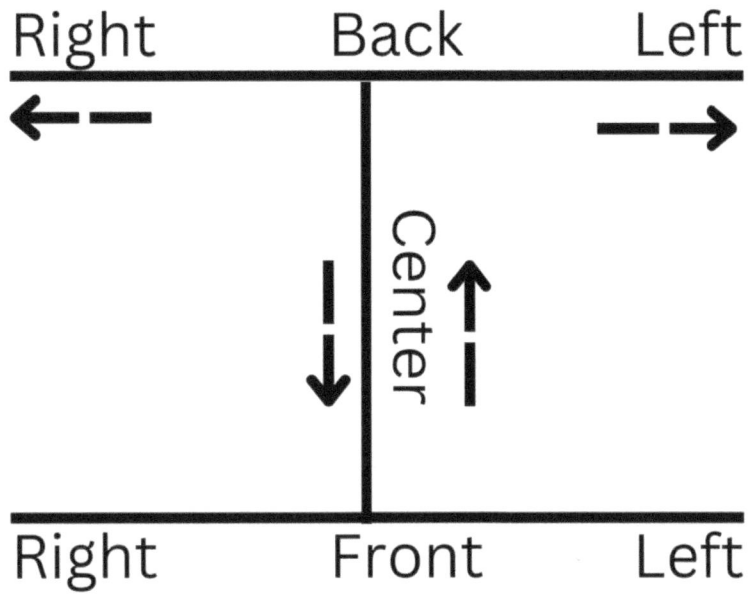

Right	Back	Left
←–		–→

Center

| Right | Front | Left |

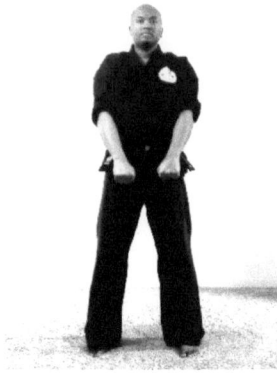

Start: Ready Stance
(Junbi Jase)

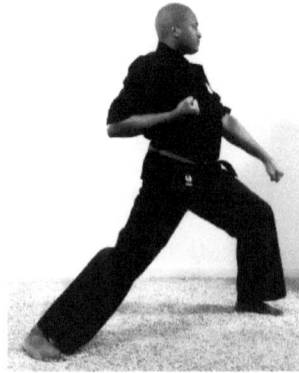

1. Turn Left 90 Degrees
Front Stance
Low Block

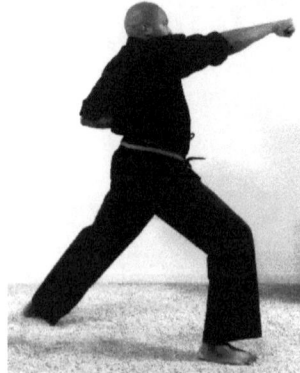

2. Step Forward
Front Stance
High Punch

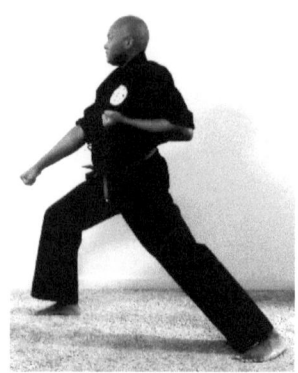

3. Turn Right 180 Degrees
Front Stance
Low Block

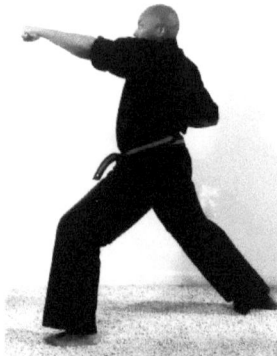

4. Step Forward
Front Stance
High Punch

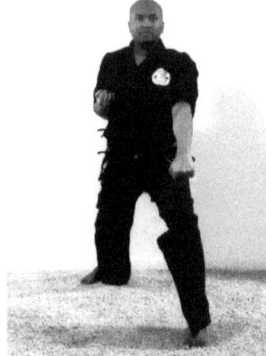

5. Turn Left 90 Degrees
Front Stance
Low Block

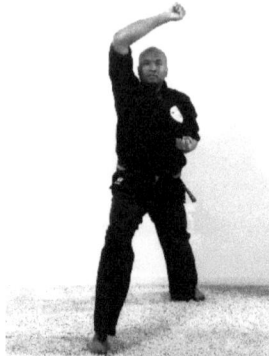

6. Step Forward
Front Stance
High Block

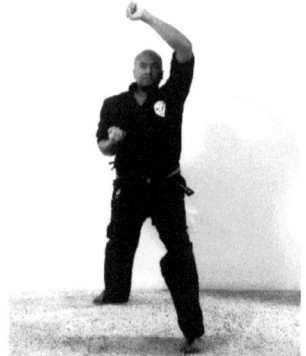

7. Step Forward
Front Stance
High Block

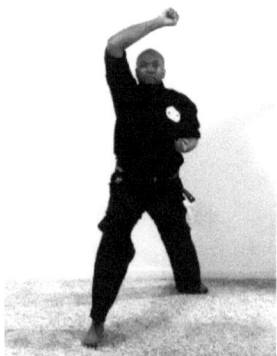

8. Step Forward
Front Stance
High Block
Kihap!

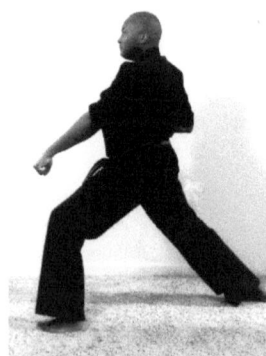

9. Turn Left 270 Degrees
Front Stance
Low Block

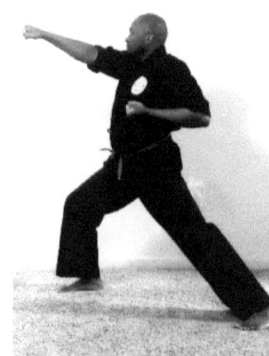

10. Step Forward
Front Stance
High Punch

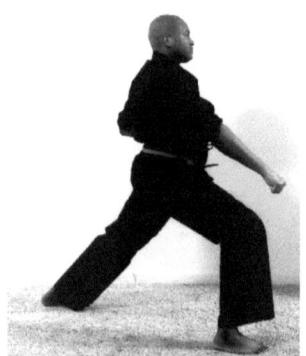

11. Turn Right 180 Degrees
Front Stance
Low Block

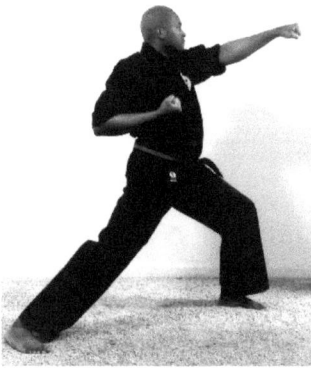

12. Step Forward
Front Stance
High Punch

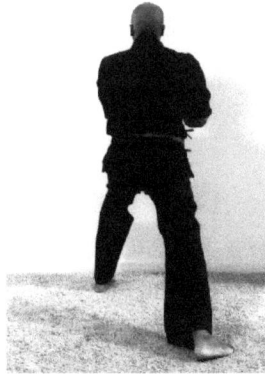

13. Turn Left 90 Degrees
Front Stance
Low Block

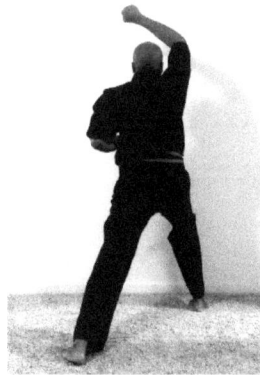

14. Step Forward
Front Stance
High Block

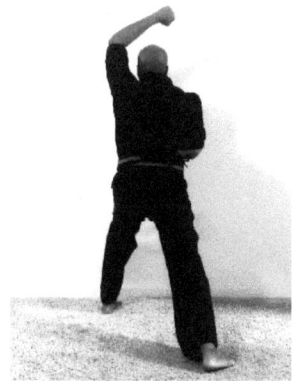

15. Step Forward
Front Stance
High Block

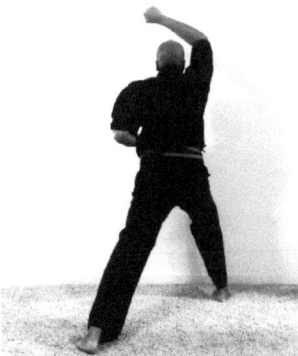

16. Step Forward
Front Stance
High Block
Kihap!

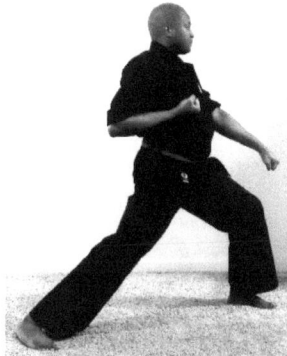

17. Turn Left 270 Degrees
Front Stance
Low Block

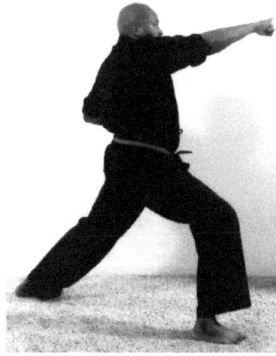

18. Step Forward
Front Stance
High Punch

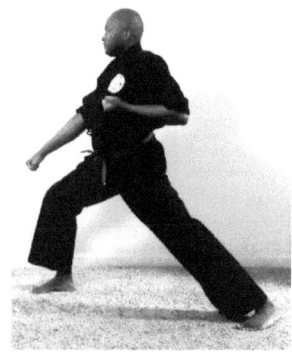

19. Turn Right 180
Degrees
Front Stance
Low Block

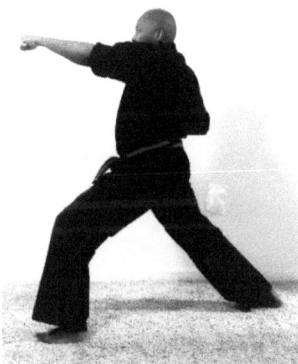

20. Step Forward
Front Stance
High Punch

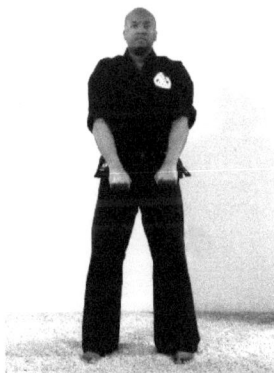

Finish: Ready Stance
(Junbi Jase)

Kicho Hyung Sahm Bu

Kicho Hyung Directions

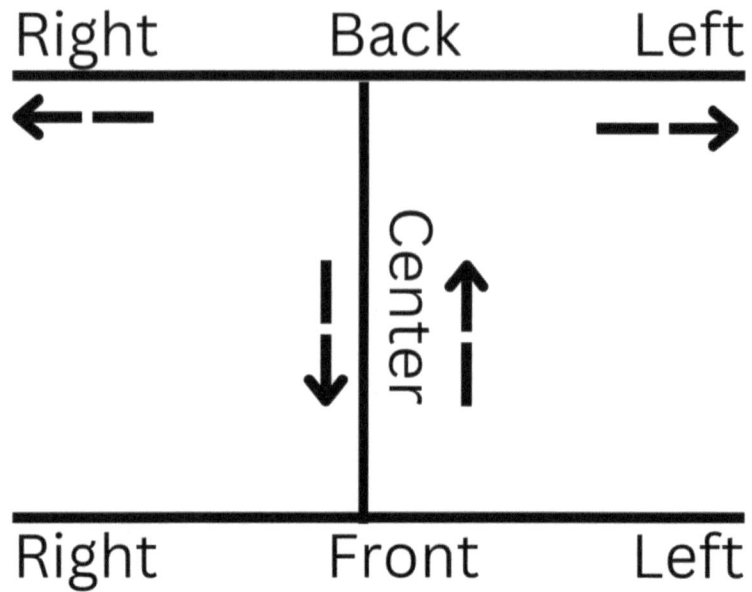

Right	Back	Left
←−	Center	−→
	↓ ↑	
Right	Front	Left

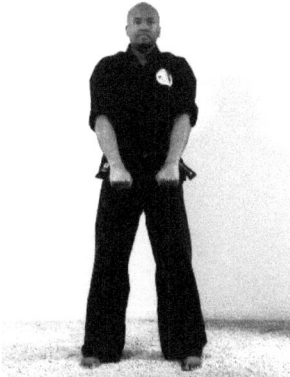

Start: Ready Stance
(Junbi Jase)

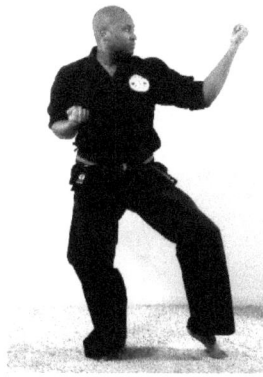

1. Turn Left 90 Degrees
Back Stance
Inside Forearm Block
_A_

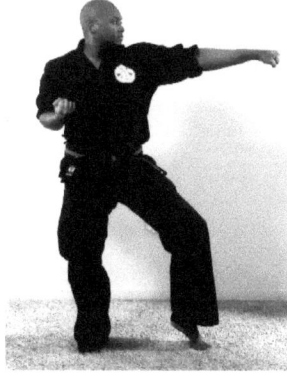

Back Stance
Push Punch
_B_

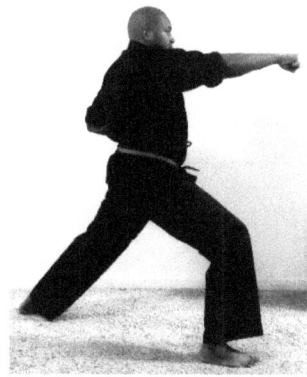

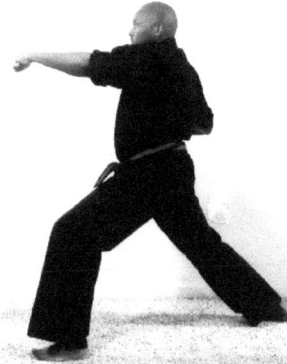

2. Step Forward
Front Stance
Middle Punch

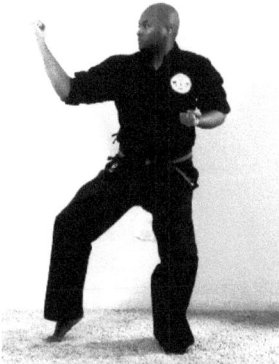

3. Turn Right 180 Degrees
Back Stance
Inside Forearm Block
_A_

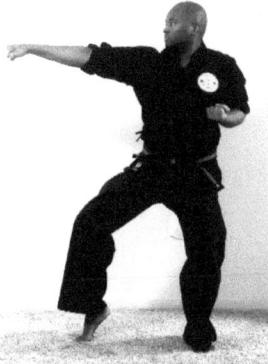

Back Stance
Push Punch
_B_

4. Step Forward
Front Stance
Middle Punch

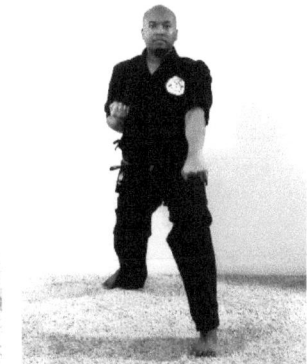

5. Turn Left 90 Degrees
Front Stance
Low Block

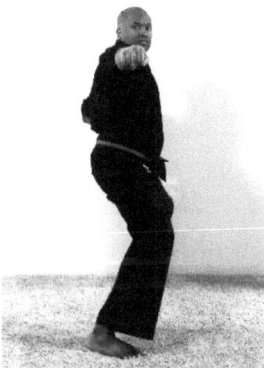

6. Step Forward
Horse Stance
Side Punch

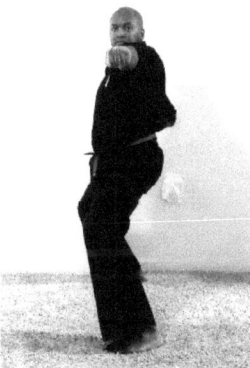

7. Step Forward
Horse Stance
Side Punch

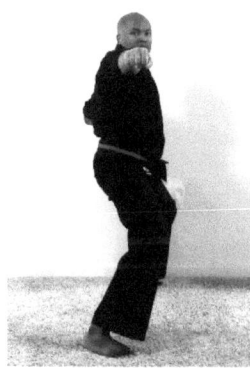

8. Step Forward
Horse Stance
Side Punch
Kihap!

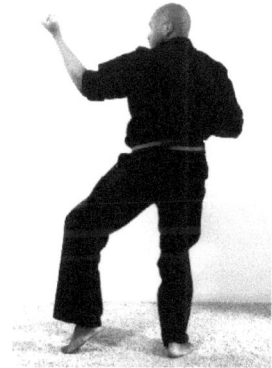

9. Turn Left 270 Degrees
Back Stance
Inside Forearm Block
_A_

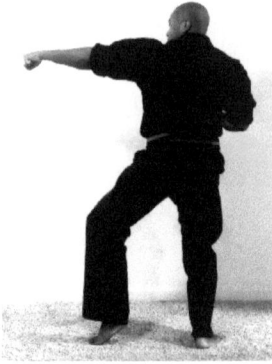

Back Stance
Push Punch
_B_

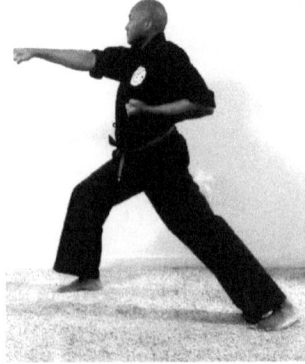

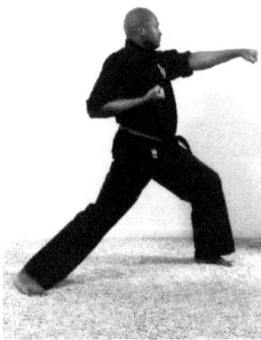

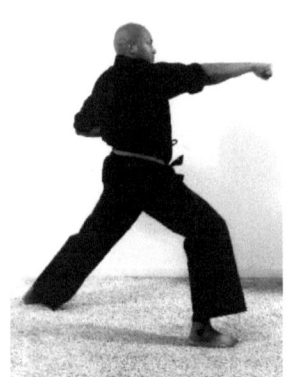

10. Step Forward
Front Stance
Middle Punch

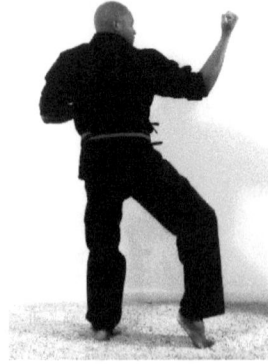

11. Turn Right 180 Degrees
Back Stance
Inside Forearm Block
_A_

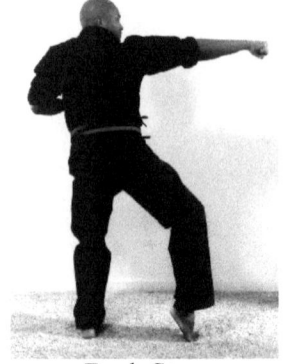

Back Stance
Push Punch
_B_

12. Step Forward
Front Stance
Middle Punch

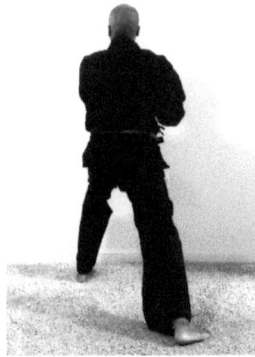

13. Turn Left 90 Degrees
Front Stance
Low Block

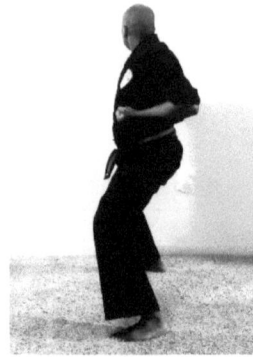

14. Step Forward
Horse Stance
Side Punch

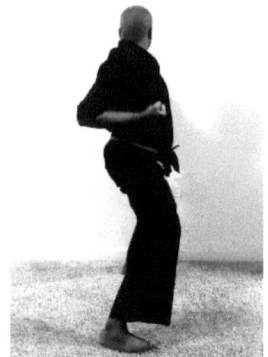

15. Step Forward
Horse Stance
Side Punch

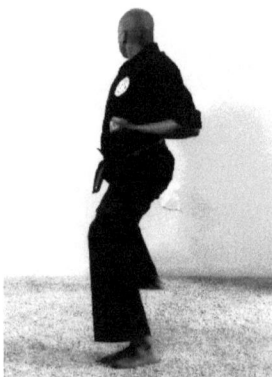

16. Step Forward
Horse Stance
Side Punch
Kihap!

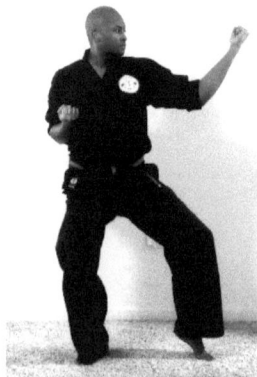

17. Turn Left 270 Degrees
Back Stance
Inside Forearm Block
_A_

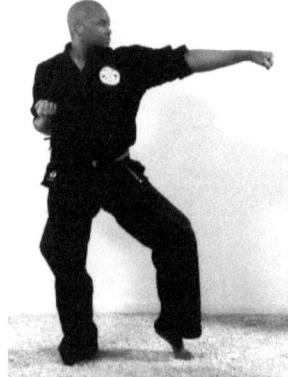

Back Stance
Push Punch
_B_

18. Step Forward
Front Stance
Middle Punch

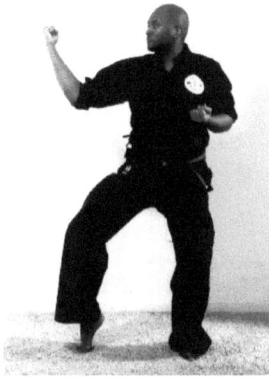

19. Turn Right 180
Degrees
Back Stance
Inside Forearm Block
A

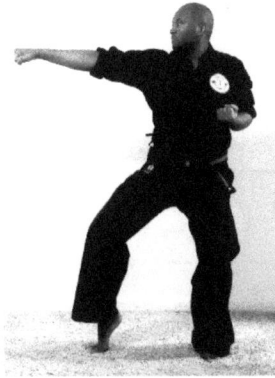

Back Stance
Push Punch
B

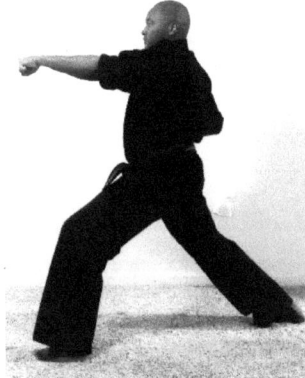

20. Step Forward
Front Stance
Middle Punch

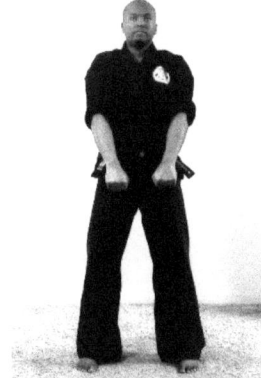

Finish: Ready Stance
(Junbi Jase)

Pyung Ahn Hyung

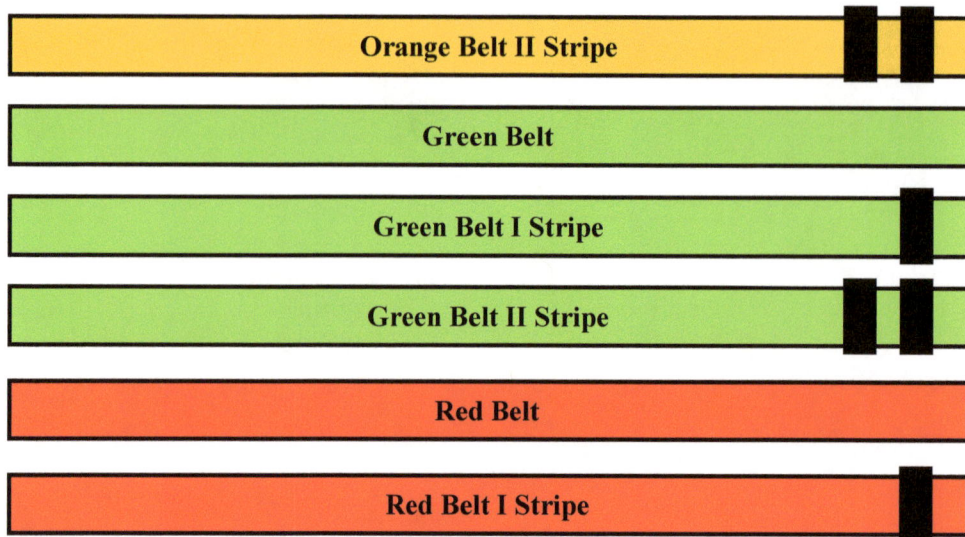

Orange Belt II Stripe	
Green Belt	
Green Belt I Stripe	
Green Belt II Stripe	
Red Belt	
Red Belt I Stripe	

The five Pyung Ahn forms are based on the five Heian kata taught in Shotokan, but with a few minor changes. They were created by Anko Itosu, an Okinawan who practiced the martial art known as Tode. They descended from one single kata known as Jae Nam (Channan). Gichin Funakoshi modified the five kata and taught them to his students.

1. Pyung Ahn Cho Dan

2. Pyung Ahn Ee Dan

3. Pyung Ahn Sahm Dan

4. Pyung Ahn Sah Dan

5. Pyung Ahn Oh Dan

Pyung Ahn Cho Dan

Pyung Ahn Cho Dan Directions

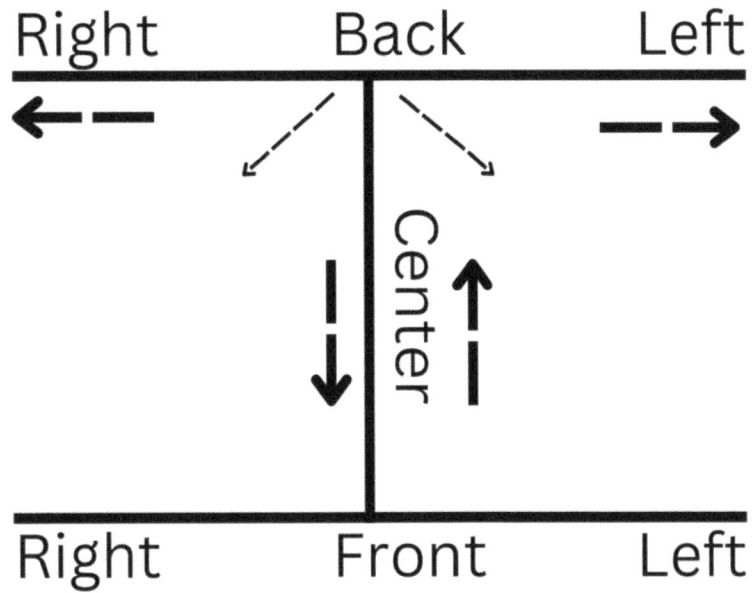

Right	Back	Left

Center

Right	Front	Left

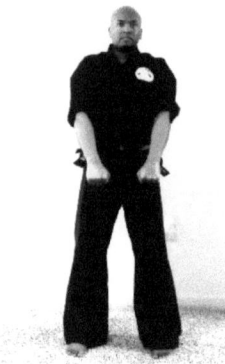

Start: Ready Stance
(Junbi Jase)

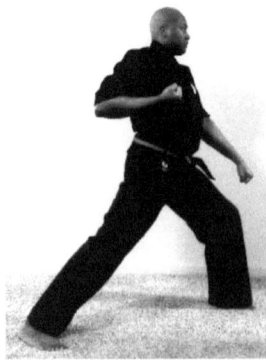

1. Turn Left 90 Degrees
Front Stance
Low Block

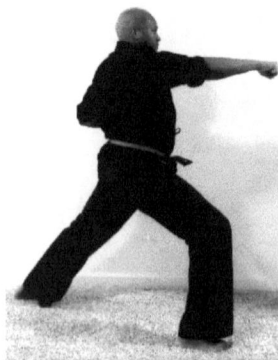

2. Step Forward
Front Stance
Middle Punch

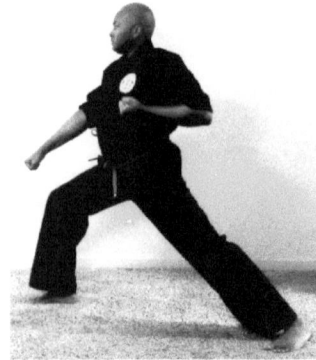

3. Turn Right 180 Degrees
Front Stance
Low Block

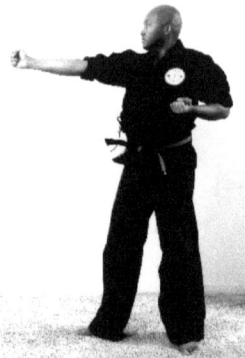

4. Perform a quick hammer
fist by bringing the right
foot to a 90-degree angle
with the left foot.

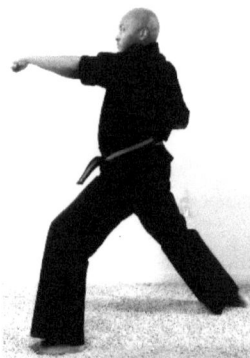

5. Step Forward
Front Stance
Middle Punch

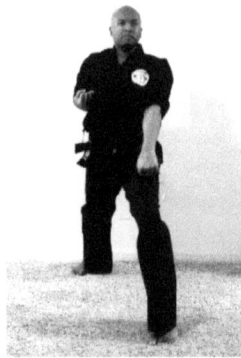

6. Turn Left 90 Degrees
Front Stance
Low Block
A

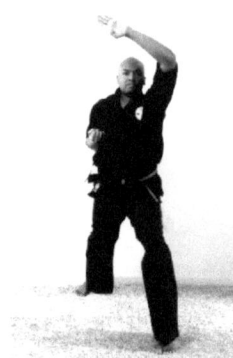

Front Stance,
Raise your left hand
above your head, as if
blocking
B

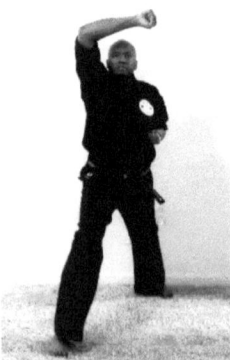

7. Step Forward
Front Stance
High Block

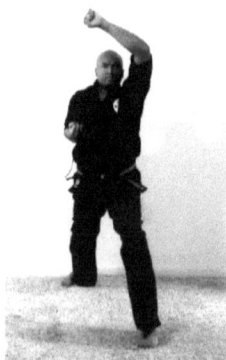

8. Step Forward
Front Stance
High Block

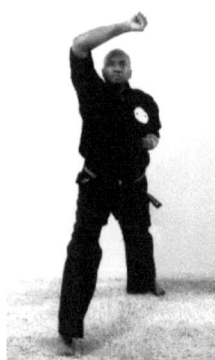

9. Step Forward
Front Stance
High Block
A

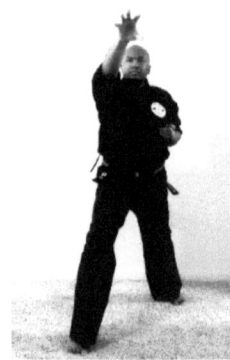

Front Stance
Hair Grab
B

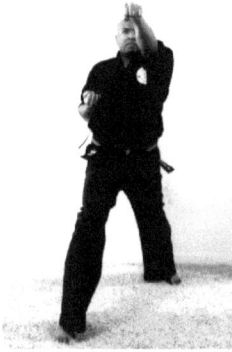

10. Front Stance
High Punch
Kihap!

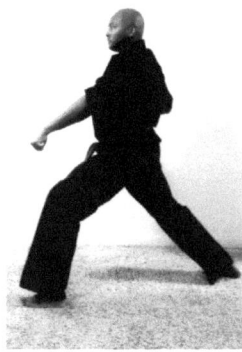

11. Turn Left 270 Degrees
Front Stance
Low Block

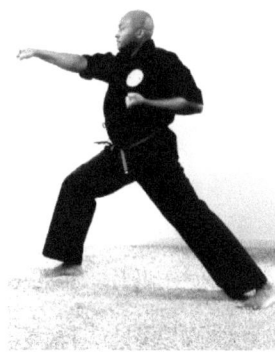

12. Step Forward
Front Stance
Middle Punch

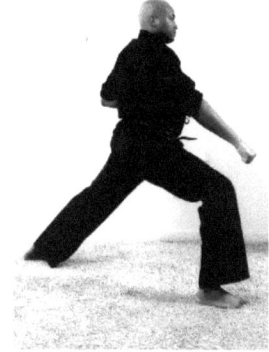

13. Turn Right 180 Degrees
Front Stance
Low Block

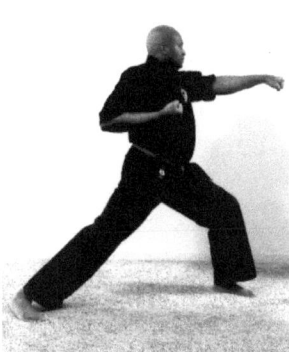

14. Step Forward
Front Stance
Middle Punch

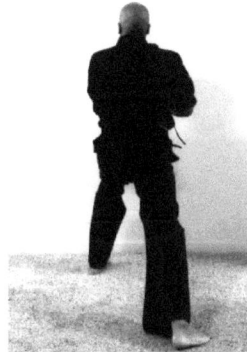

15. Turn Left 90 Degrees
Front Stance
Low Block

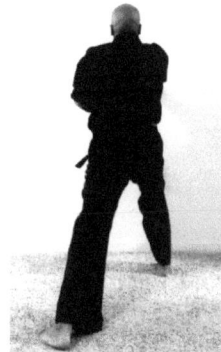

16. Step Forward
Front Stance
Middle Punch

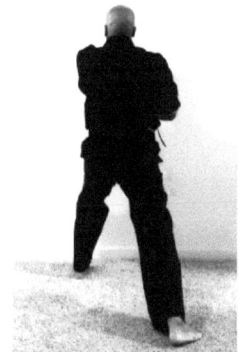

17. Step Forward
Front Stance
Middle Punch

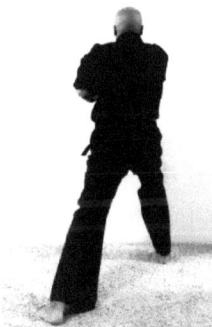

18. Step Forward
Front Stance
Middle Punch
Kihap!

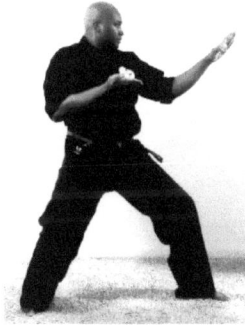

19. Turn Left 270 Degrees
Back Stance
Double Knifehand Block

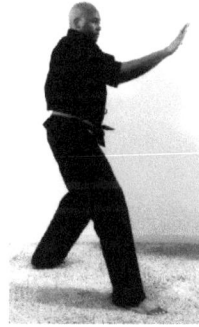

20. Using your right foot,
turn right at 45 degrees.
Back Stance
Double Knifehand Block

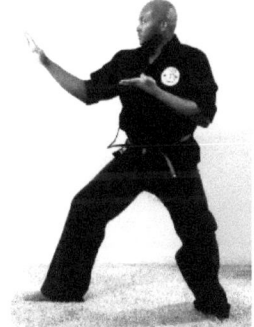

21. Turn Right 135 Degrees
Back Stance
Double Knifehand Block

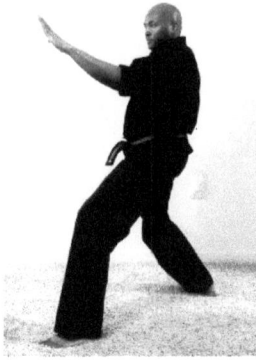

22. Using your left foot, turn left at 45 degrees.
Back Stance
Double Knifehand Block

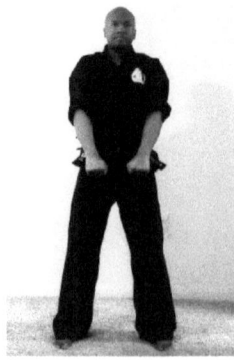

Finish: Ready Stance (Junbi Jase)

Pyung Ahn Ee Dan

Pyung Ahn Ee Dan Directions

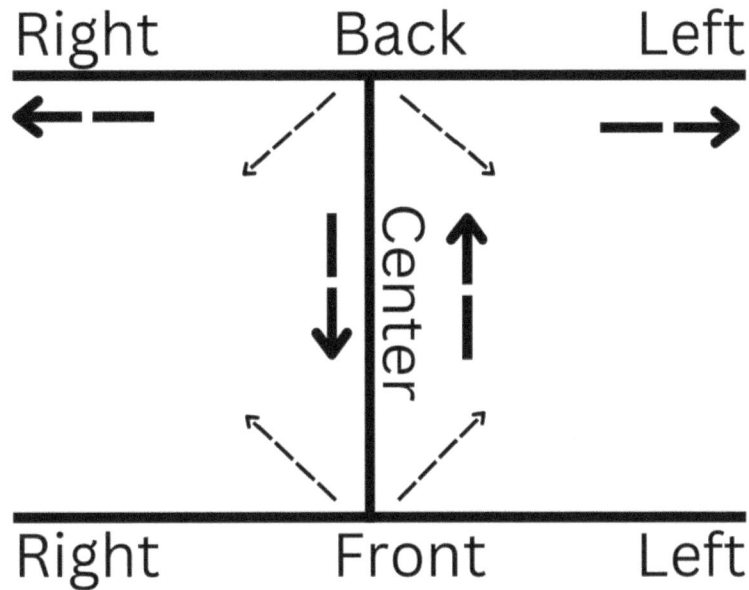

Right	Back	Left
← -		- →

Center

| Right | Front | Left |

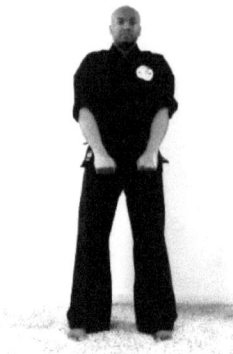

Start: Ready Stance
(Junbi Jase)

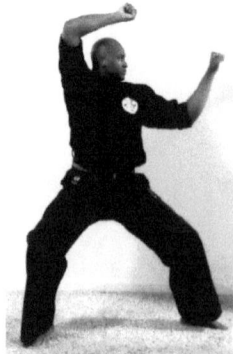

1. Turn Left 90 Degrees
Back Stance
Twin Forearm Block
A

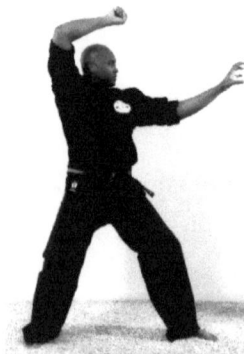

Back Stance
Lapel Grab
B

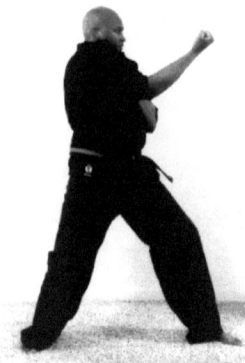

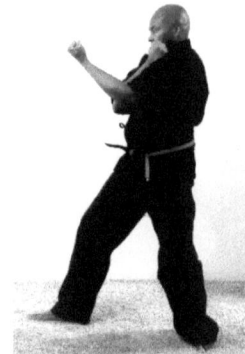

2. Back Stance
Hammerfist to Jaw

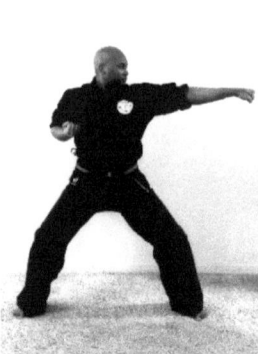

3. Horse Stance
Side Punch

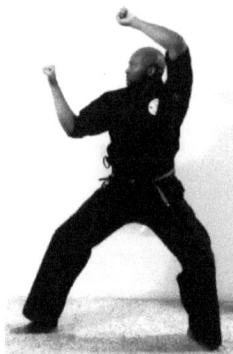

4. Turn Right 180 Degrees
Back Stance
Twin Forearm Block
A

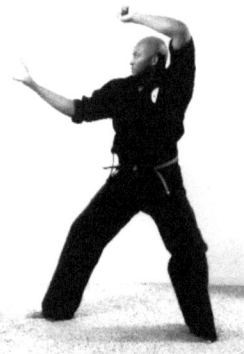

Back Stance
Lapel Grab
B

5. Back Stance
Hammerfist to Jaw

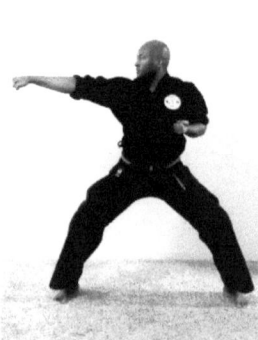

6. Horse Stance
Side Punch

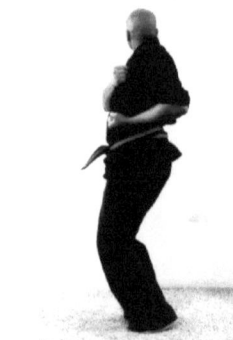

7. Move the right foot
toward the left foot while
looking back with both
fists on the left side.

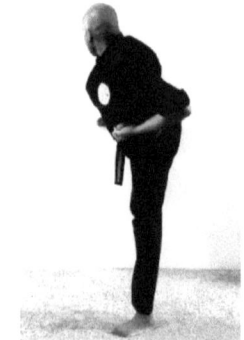

8. Perform a backfist and
side kick with your right
side at the same time.

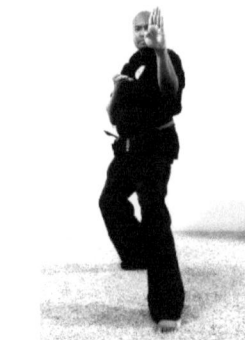

9. Turn Left 180 Degrees
Back Stance
Double Knifehand Block

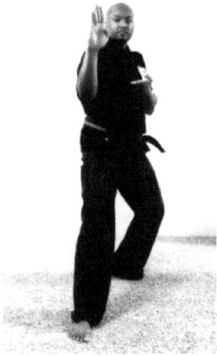

10. Step Forward
Back Stance
Double Knifehand Block

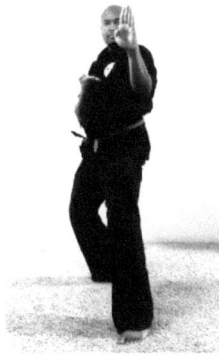

11. Step Forward
Back Stance
Double Knifehand Block

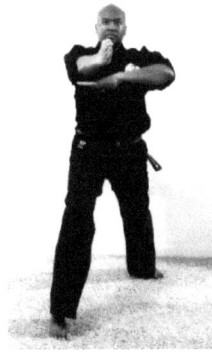

12. Step Forward
Front Stance
Spear Hand
Kihap!

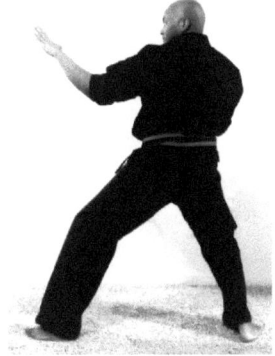

13. Turn Left 270 Degrees
Back Stance
Double Knifehand Block

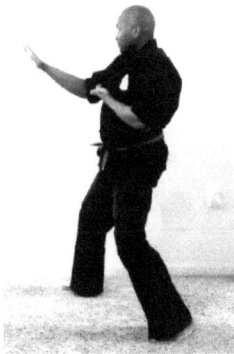

14. Turn Right 45 Degrees
Back Stance
Double Knifehand Block

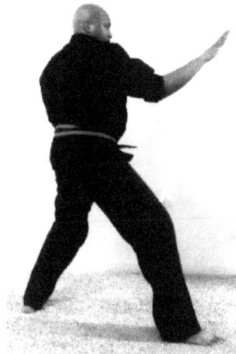

15. Turn Right 135 Degrees
Back Stance
Double Knifehand Block

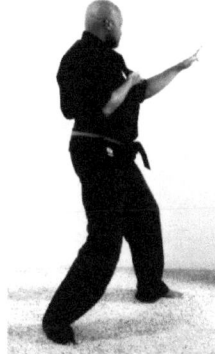

16. Turn Left 45 Degrees
Back Stance
Double Knifehand Block

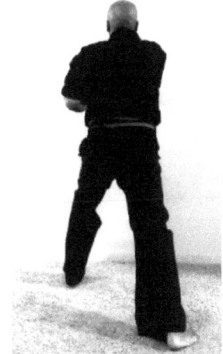

17. Turn left 45 Degrees
Front Stance
With your right arm,
middle punch an
inside block.

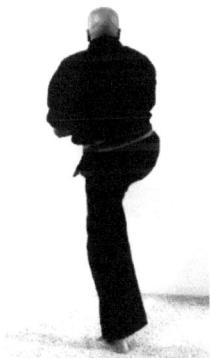

18. Use your right foot to
perform a Front kick.

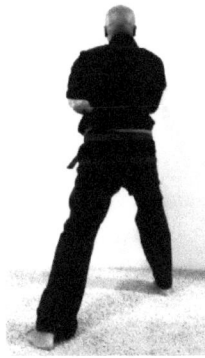

19. Step Forward
Front Stance
With your left arm,
middle punch an
inside block.

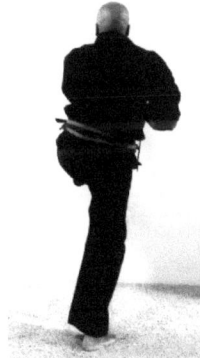

20. Use your left foot to
perform a Front kick.

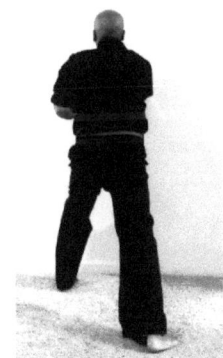

21. Step Forward
Front Stance
perform a middle punch
with your right arm.
Kihap!

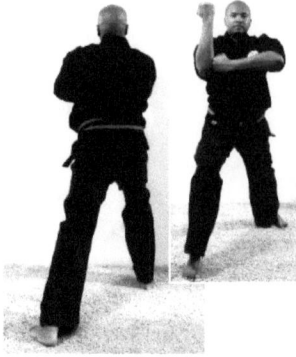

22. Step Forward
Front Stance
Double Forearm Block

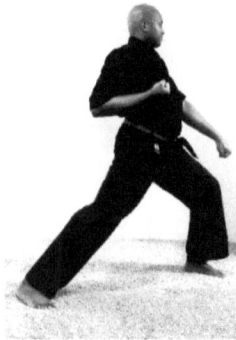

23. Turn Left 270 Degrees
Front Stance
Low Block
A

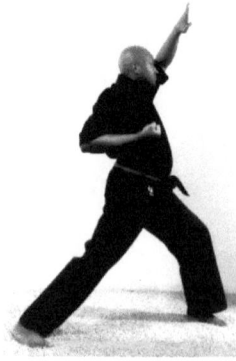

Front Stance,
Raise your left hand
above your head, as if
blocking
B

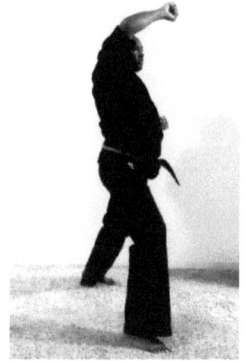

24. Turn Right 45 Degrees
Front Stance
Hight Block

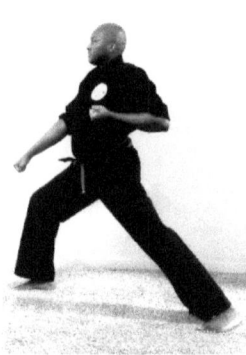

25. Turn Left 180 Degrees
Front Stance
Low Block
A

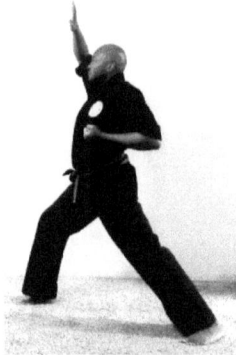

Front Stance,
Raise your right hand
above your head, as if
blocking
B

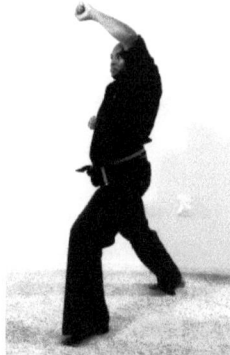

26. Turn Right 45 Degrees
Front Stance
Hight Block

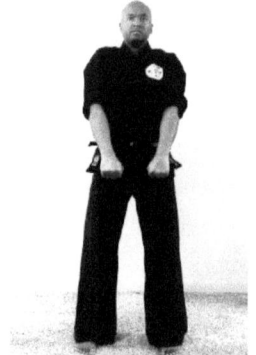

Finish: Ready Stance
(Junbi Jase)

Pyung Ahn Sahm Dan

Pyung Ahn Sahm Dan Directions

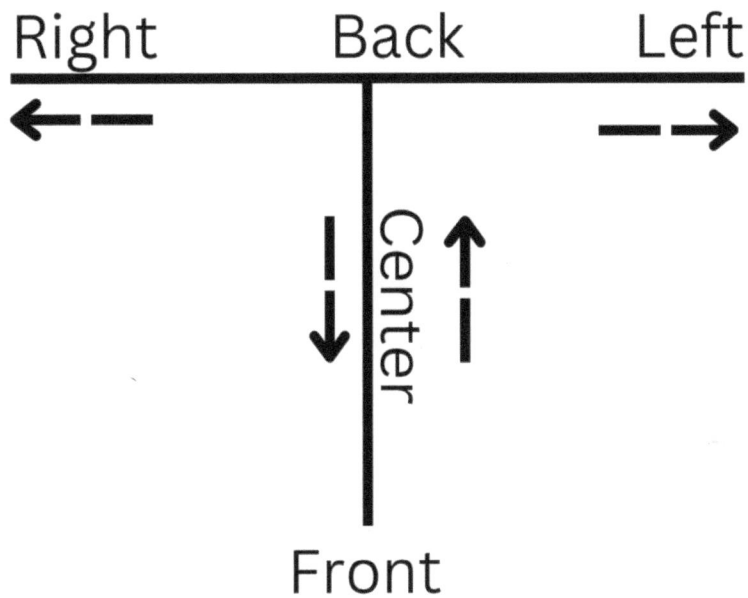

Right   Back   Left

← –   → →

↓   ↑
Center

Front

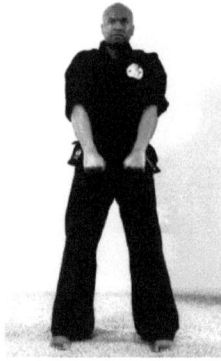

Start: Ready Stance (Junbi Jase)

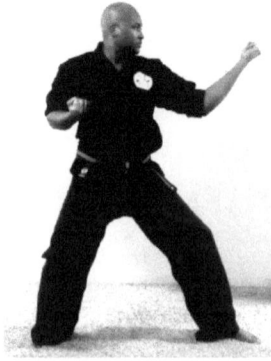

1. Turn Left 90 Degrees Back Stance Twin Forearm Block

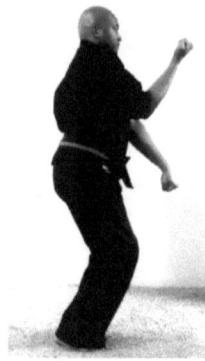

2. Perform an inside block with the right arm and a low block with the left arm simultaneously. Shift the right foot next to the left foot, bringing the feet together.

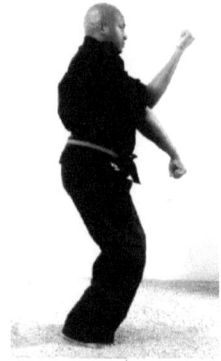

3. While keeping both feet together, simultaneously execute a low block with the right arm and an inside block with the left arm.

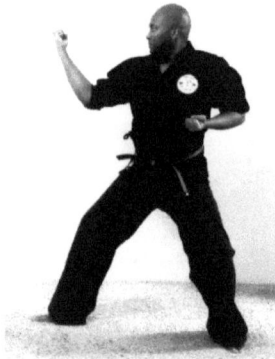

4. Turn Right 180 Degrees Back Stance Twin Forearm Block

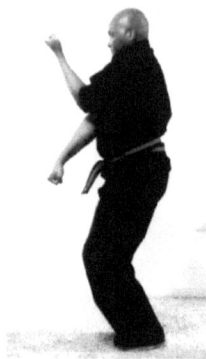

5. Perform an inside block with the left arm and a low block with the right arm simultaneously. Shift the left foot next to the right foot, bringing the feet together.

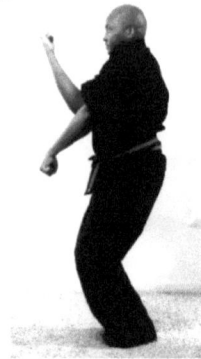

6. While keeping both feet together, simultaneously execute a low block with the left arm and an inside block with the right arm.

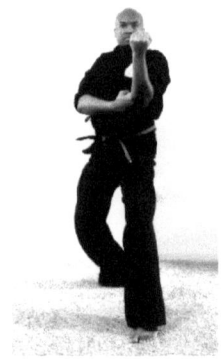

7. Turn left 90 Degrees Back Stance Double Forearm Block

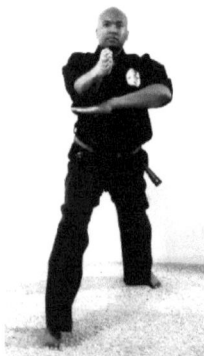

8. Step Forward Front Stance Spear Hand

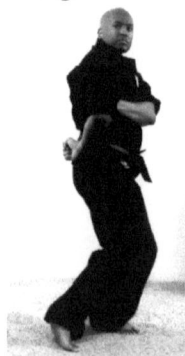

9. Looking forward, slightly bend your elbow and move your right hand to your right waist. Take a large step forward, placing your left leg behind your right, forming a cross stance.

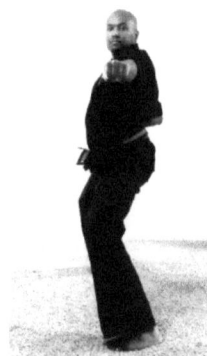

10. Make a left-handed hammer fist strike as you turn left into a horse stance.

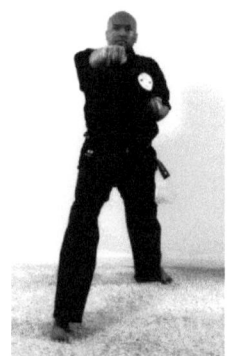

11. Step Forward Front Stance Middle Punch Kihap!

28

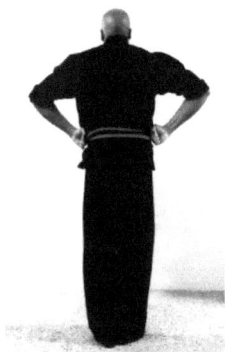

12. As you turn 180 degrees to the left to face the opposite direction, bring the left foot in line with the right foot. Put both of your hands on your waist.

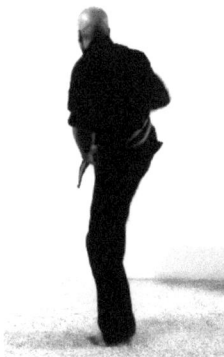

13. Use your right foot to perform an inside crescent kick.

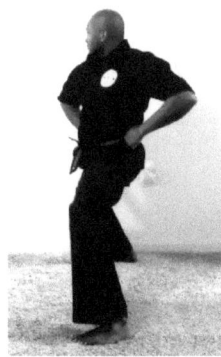

14. Horse Stance Elbow Block

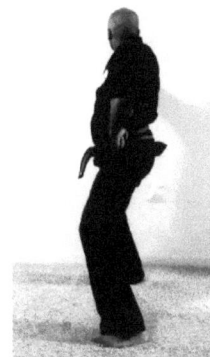

15. Horse Stance Backfist

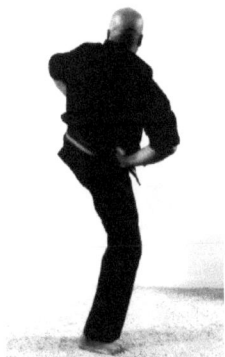

16. Use your left foot to perform an inside crescent kick.

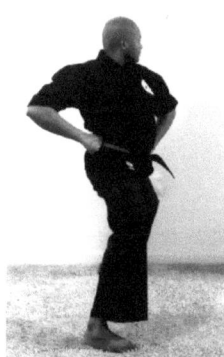

17. Horse Stance Elbow Block

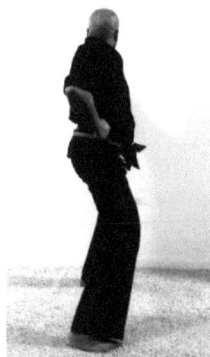

18. Horse Stance Backfist

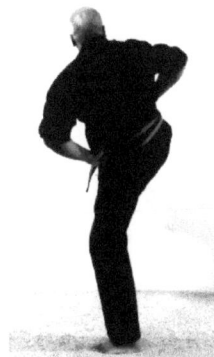

19. Use your right foot to perform an inside crescent kick.

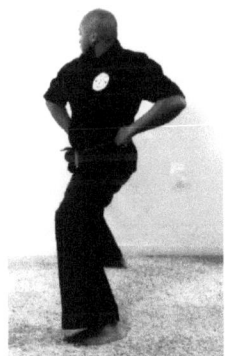

20. Horse Stance Elbow Block

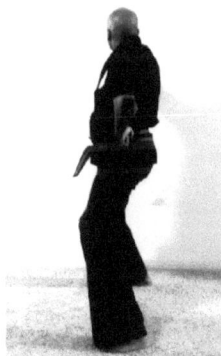

21. Horse Stance Backfist

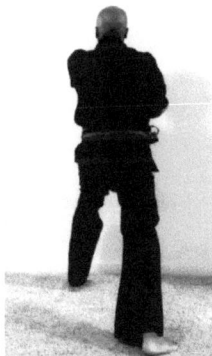

22. Step Forward with your left foot into a Front Stance, Middle Punch Kihap!

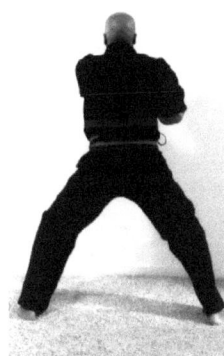

23. Bring the right foot in line with the left foot.

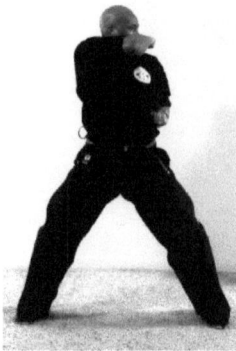

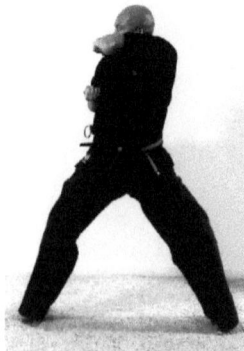

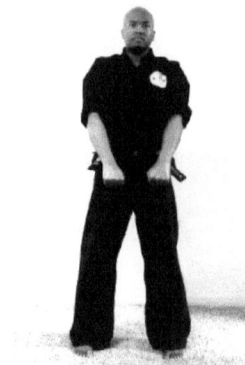

24. Turn 180 degrees to the left into a horse stance, punch over your left shoulder, and strike with your left elbow at the same time.

25. Jump to your right in a horse stance, punch over your right shoulder and strike with your right elbow at the same time.

Finish: Ready Stance (Junbi Jase)

Pyung Ahn Sah Dan

Pyung Ahn Sah Dan Directions

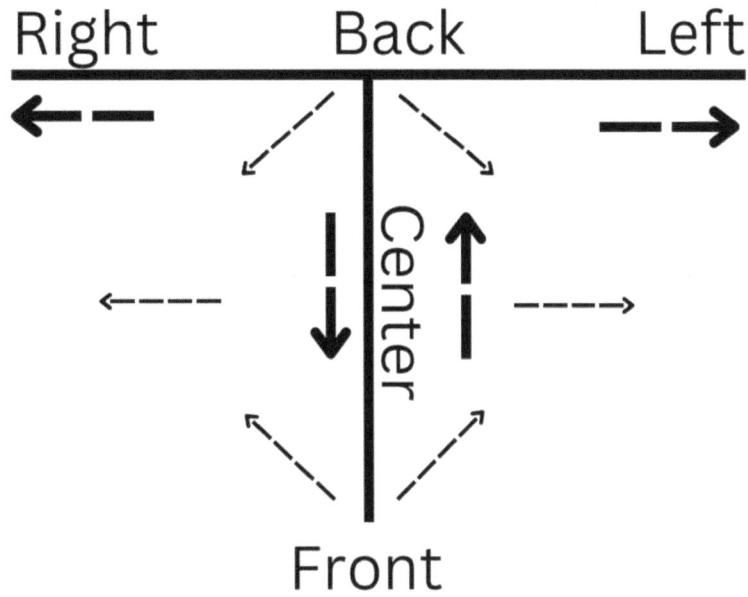

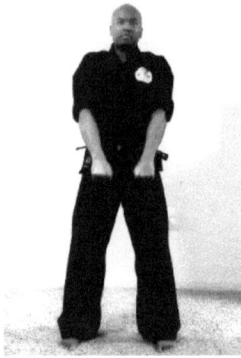

Start: Ready Stance
(Junbi Jase)

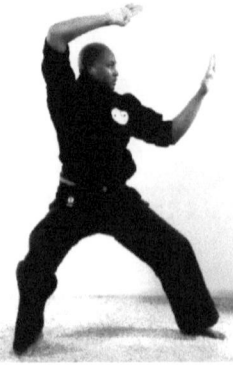

1. Turn Left 90 Degrees
Back Stance
Twin Knifehand Block

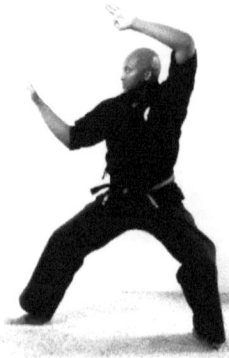

2. Turn Right 180 Degrees
Back Stance
Twin Knifehand Block

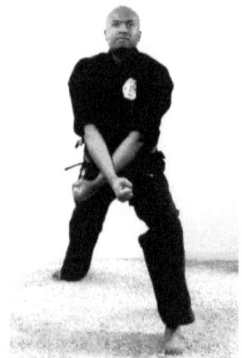

3. Turn Left 90 Degrees
Front Stance
Low X Block

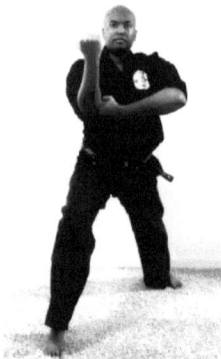

4. Step Forward
Front Stance
Double Forearm Block

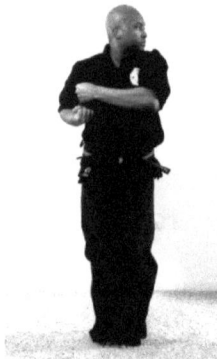

5. Place both fists to the right as you turn left 90 degrees and bring your feet together.

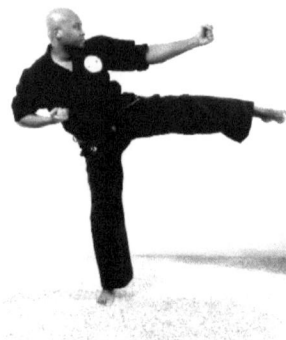

6. Perform both a backfist and a side kick at the same time.

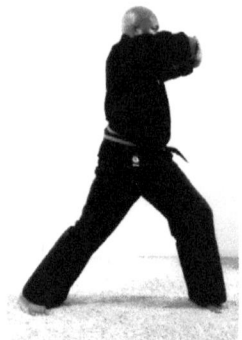

7. Take a forward step into a front stance. Strike your left palm with your right elbow.

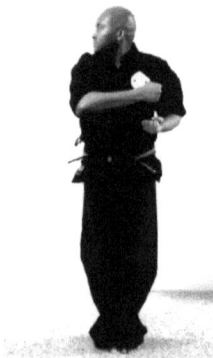

8. Place both fists to the left as you turn right 180 degrees and bring your feet together.

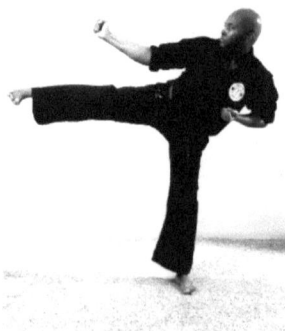

9. Perform both a backfist and a side kick at the same time.

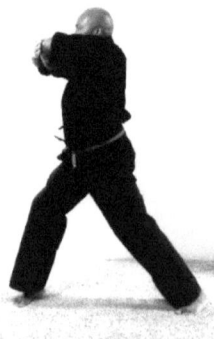

10. Take a forward step into a front stance. Strike your right palm with your left elbow.

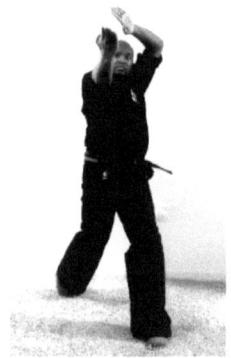

11. While pivoting on both feet with the left foot pointing forward and turning left 90 degrees, perform a high knifehand block with your left hand and a chop with your right hand.

32

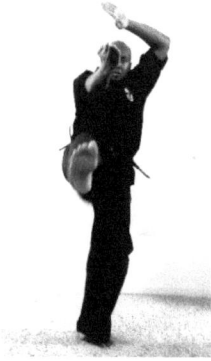

12. Perform a front kick with your right foot.

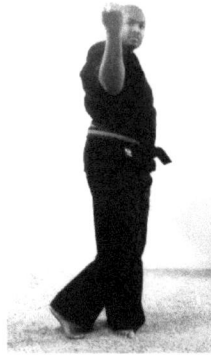

13. Perform a backfist with your right hand as you leap forward and place your left leg behind your right in a cross stance. Kihap!

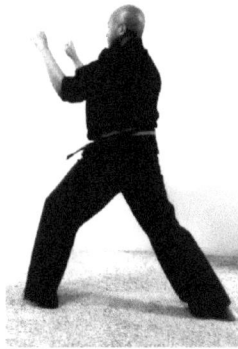

14. Turn left 135 degrees into a front stance and perform a high outer forearm wedging block.

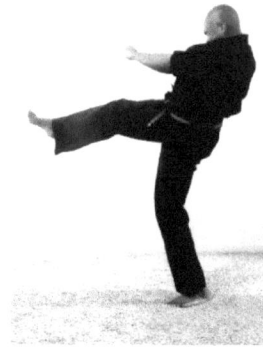

15. Keep your left fist raised as a push punch while performing a front kick with your right foot.

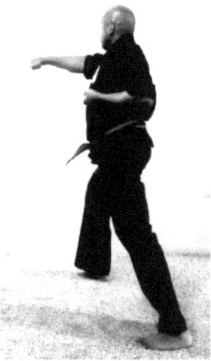

16. Perform a middle punch with your right hand as you step forward into a front stance with your right foot.

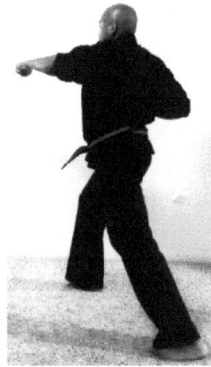

17. Perform a middle punch with your left hand.

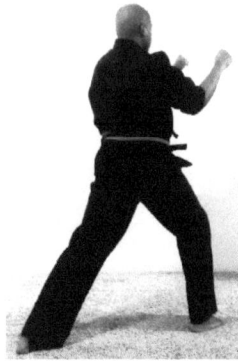

18. Turn right 90 degrees into a front stance and perform a high outer forearm wedging block.

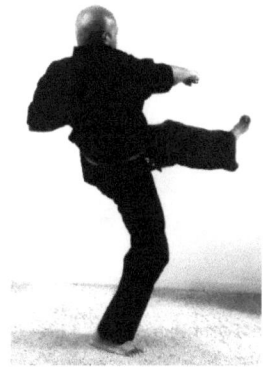

19. Keep your right fist raised as a push punch while performing a front kick with your left foot.

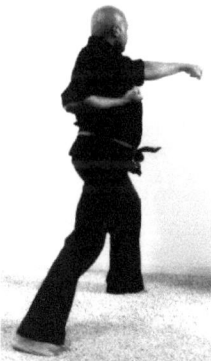

20. Perform a middle punch with your left hand as you step forward into a front stance with your left foot.

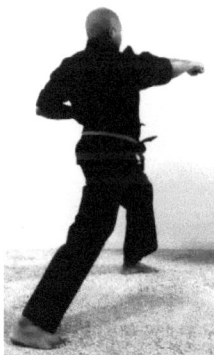

21. Perform a middle punch with your right hand.

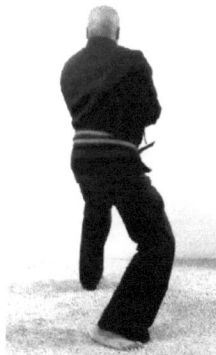

22. Turn left into a back stance, place the left foot forward, and perform a double forearm block.

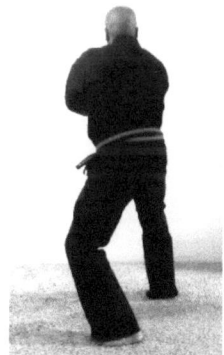

23. Step Forward Back Stance Double Forearm Block

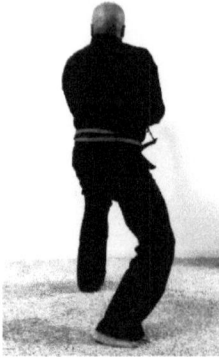

24. Step Forward
Back Stance
Double Forearm Block

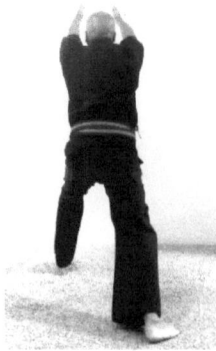

25. Shift forward into a front stance while keeping your left foot in front, and raise both of your open hands to the level of your neck.

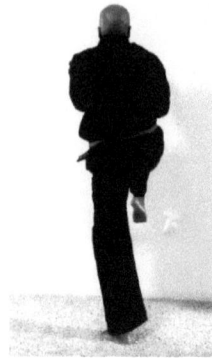

26. Strike with the right knee and pull both hands down beside the knee. Kihap!

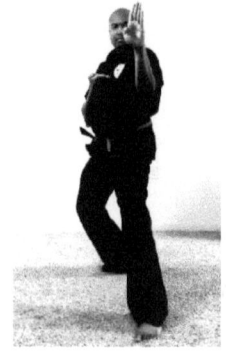

27. Turn Left 180 Degrees
Back Stance
Double Knifehand Block

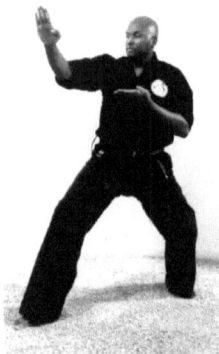

28. In a back stance, make a 45-degree turn to the right, step forward with your right foot, and double knifehand block.

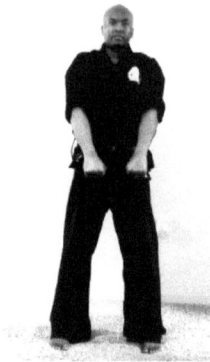

Finish: Ready Stance (Junbi Jase)

Pyung Ahn Oh Dan

Pyung Ahn Oh Dan Directions

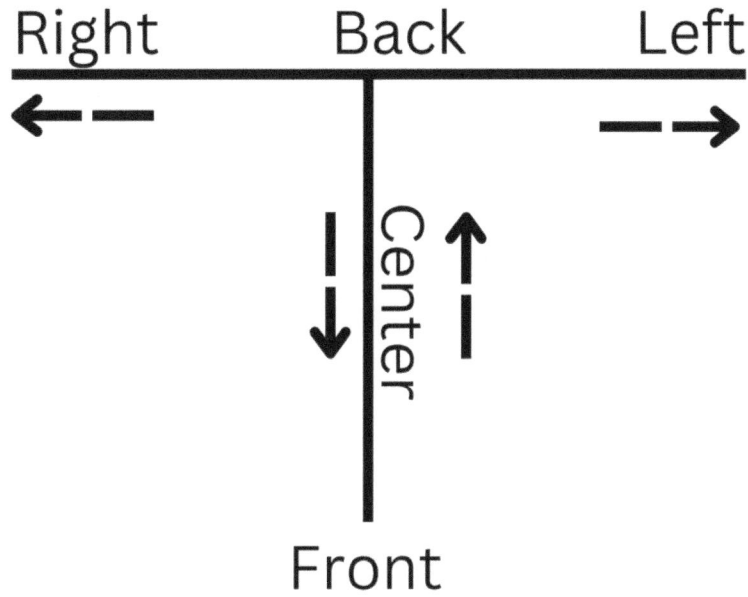

Right Back Left

Center

Front

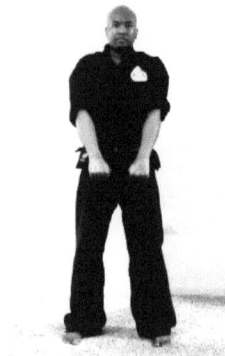

Start: Ready Stance
(Junbi Jase)

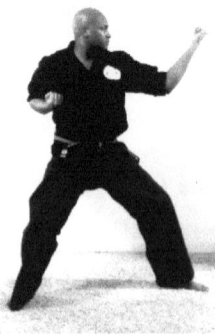

1. Turn Left 90 Degrees
Back Stance
Inside Forearm Block

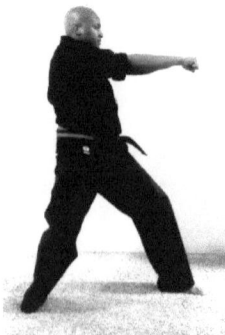

2. While in a back stance, perform a reverse middle punch with your right arm.

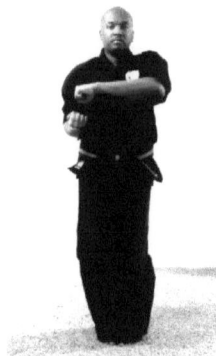

3. Bring your right foot to the side of your left foot as you turn 90 degrees to the right. Place both of your fists to the right.

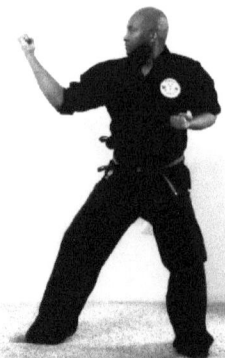

4. Turn Right 90 Degrees
Back Stance
Inside Forearm Block

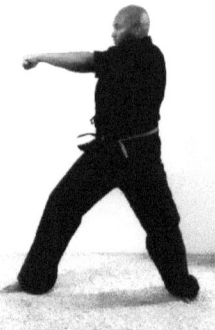

5. While in a back stance, perform a reverse middle punch with your left arm.

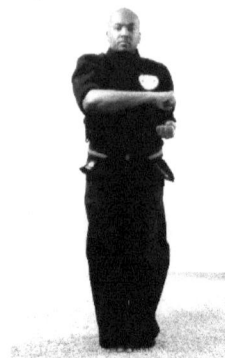

6. Bring your left foot to the side of your right foot as you turn 90 degrees to the left. Place both of your fists to the left.

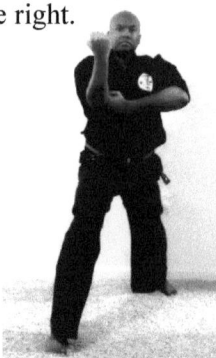

7. Step forward with your right foot into a front stance and perform a double forearm block.

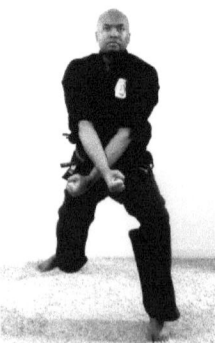

8. Step Forward
Front Stance
Low X Block

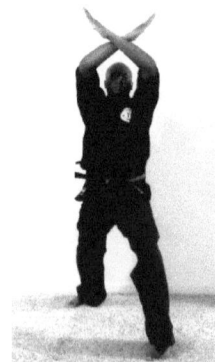

9. Front Stance
High X Block

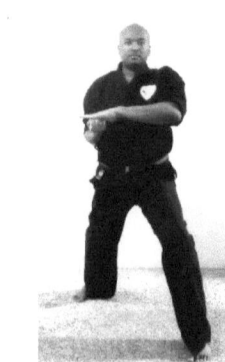

10. Move both of your hands to the right side of your waist. Keep your left hand open while making a fist with your right hand.

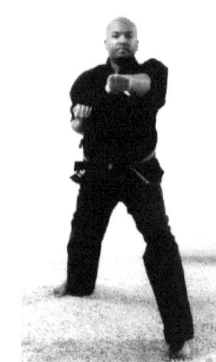

11. Perform a middle push punch with the left hand while in a front stance.

36

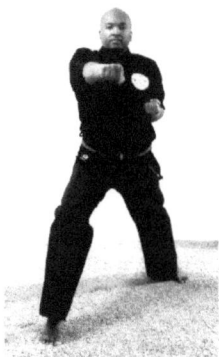

12. Step Forward Front Stance Middle Punch Kihap!

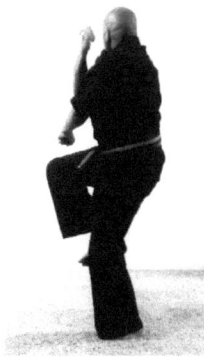

13. Cross both arms in front of your body, face the rear, and balance on the left leg.

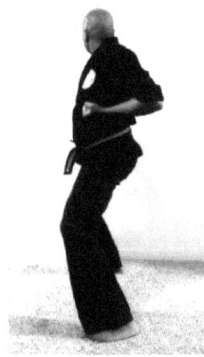

14. As you fall into a horse stance with your right foot, perform a low block with your right arm.

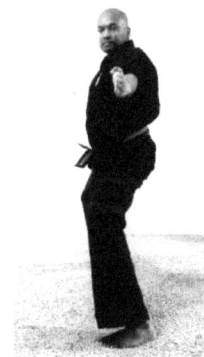

15. Turn 180 degrees to the left. Horse stance: extended left arm, open hand.

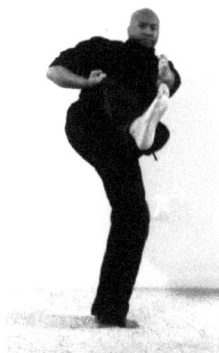

16. Strike your left open palm with your right foot, using an inside crescent kick.

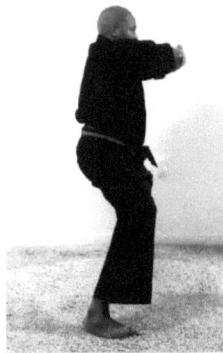

17. Strike your left open palm with your right elbow as you stamp down into a horse stance with the right foot.

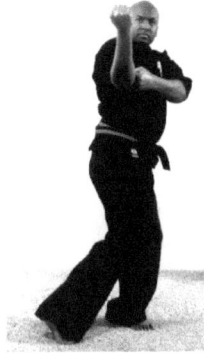

18. Turn your head 90 degrees to the right and take a large step forward, placing your left leg behind your right, forming a cross stance. Perform a double forearm block.

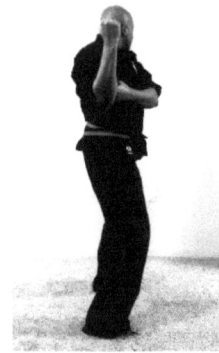

19. Turn 180 degrees to the left and bring your feet together.

A

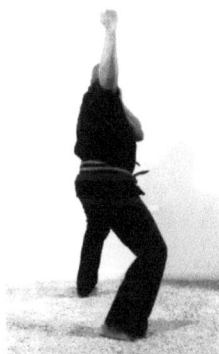

Straighten your right arm while maintaining the same posture with your left arm as you transition into a back stance.

B

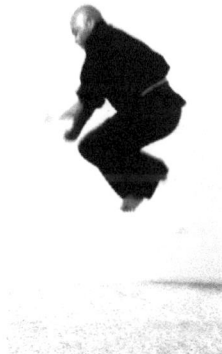

20. Jump forward into a cross stance and turn 180 degrees as you do a low X block.

A

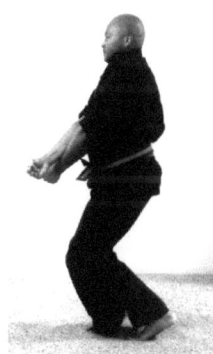

Cross Stance
Low X Block

B

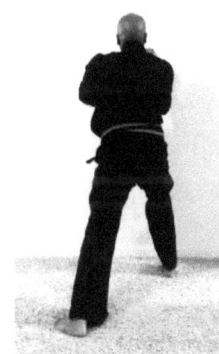

21. Step Forward Front Stance Double Forearm Block

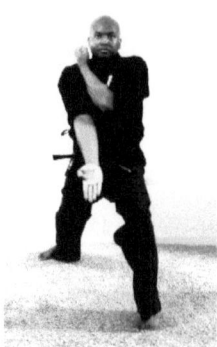

22. Turn left 180 degrees into a front stance and perform a low spear hand with your right hand while bringing your left hand beside your right ear.

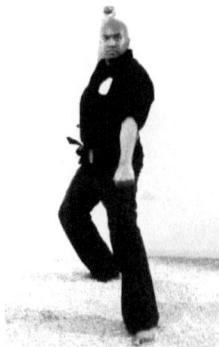

23. Shift into a back stance and pull your right arm behind you into an inside block while performing a low block with the left arm.

__A__

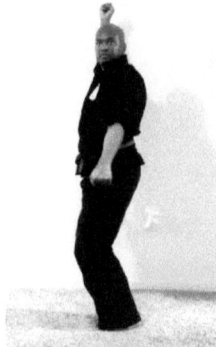

Bring your feet together by bringing your left foot to the side of your right foot.

__B__

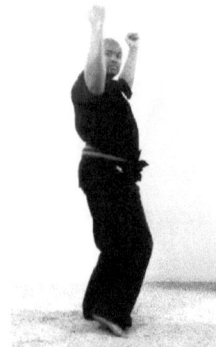

24. Turn left 180 degrees into a cross stance and perform a mountain block.

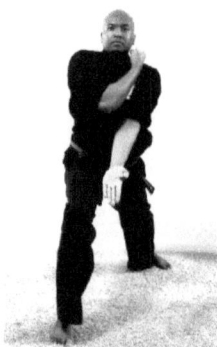

25. Turn right 90 degrees into a front stance and perform a low spear hand with your left hand while bringing your right hand beside your left ear.

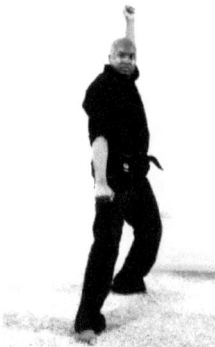

26. Shift into a back stance and pull your left arm behind you into an inside block while performing a low block with the right arm.
Kihap!

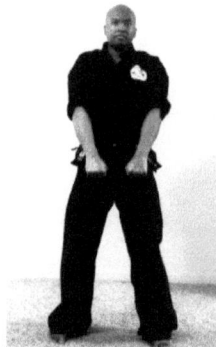

Finish: Ready Stance (Junbi Jase)

Bassai Hyung

"Passai," which is also spelled "Bassai," refers to a set of kata that are used in a variety of martial arts styles, including Korean martial arts such as Taekwondo, Tang Soo Do, and Soo Bahk Do. Although Gichin Funakoshi initially spelled the name of this form as "Passai," the kata are generally referred to as "Bassai" in Japanese styles of karate and "Passai" in Okinawan styles. The kata have a number of names in Korean: Bal Sak, Bal Sae, Ba Sa Hee, Pal Che, Palsek, and Bassahee.

Many cultures, including China, the Ryukyu Islands, Japan, and Korea, have practiced this kata. There are a number of theories regarding this kata's past, despite the fact that its origins are unknown. Some academics believe the Passai kata is related to the Chinese Leopard and Lion Boxing forms. Some sequences are similar to those in leopard boxing, such as the initial blocking and striking movement in a cross-legged posture, while others are similar to those in lion boxing, such as open-handed techniques and stomping actions. According to Okinawan karate researcher Akio Kinjo, the word comes from the Chinese word "bàosh," which means "leopard-lion" and is spelled "Bá-săi" or "pà-sai" in some dialects of Chinese.

Some Chinese origin theorists also believe that this style is a representation of the Wuxing Quan style of kung fu, also known as the "five-element fist style." Other theories believe that Passai, like other mainstream kata, was a component of the Crane Boxing System, which had a significant impact on Okinawan karate. Given that the majority of the katas are based on or adaptations of forms from the Fukien Crane style, this may appear to be a very obvious conclusion. However, many Chinese styles and Okinawan instructors were influenced by the Fujian white crane style.

The older the version of Passai, the more Chinese links make sense. Unfortunately, because it is not particularly practiced in modern China, Passai's actual lineage may never be determined.

Bassai

Bassai Directions

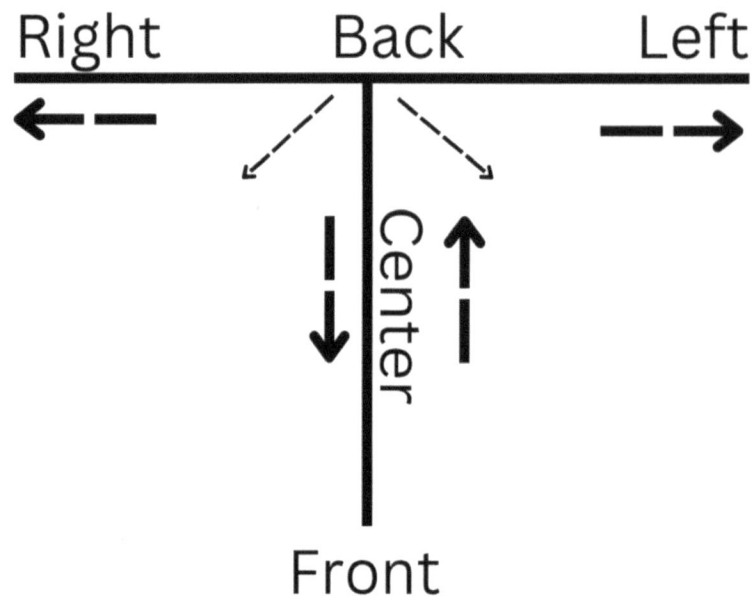

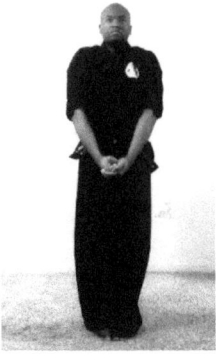

Start: Ready Stance
(Bassai)

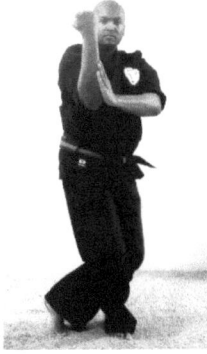

1. Step forward and turn 90 degrees to the left, placing your left leg behind your right, forming a cross stance. Keep your left hand open and perform a double forearm block.

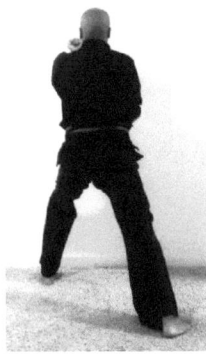

2. Turn 180 degrees to the left. In a front stance with the left foot forward, quickly execute an inside block with the right arm and an outside block with the left arm.

3. In a front stance with the left foot forward, quickly execute an inside block with the left arm and an outside block with the right arm.

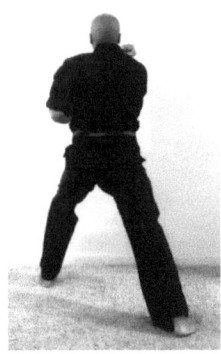

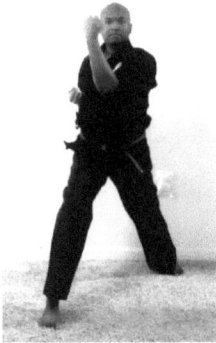

4. Turn 180 degrees to the right. In a front stance with the right foot forward, quickly execute an inside block with the left arm.

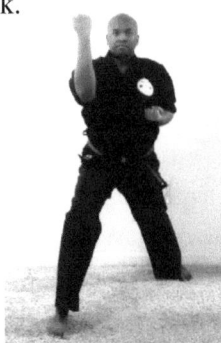

5. Quickly execute an outside block with the right arm.

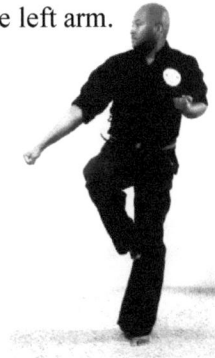

6. Perform a low block with your right arm as you turn 90 degrees to the right and balance on your left leg.

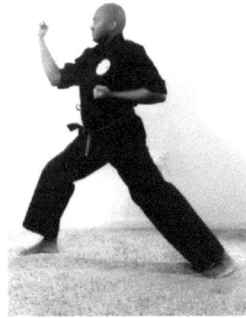

7. Turn Right 90 Degrees
Front Stance
Inside Block (R)

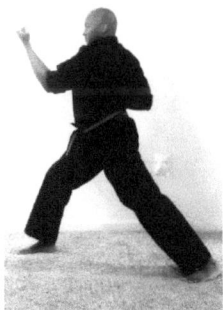

8. Front Stance
Outside Block (L)

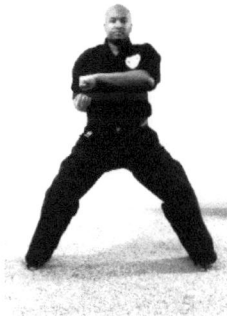

9. Shift into a horse stance while turning 90 degrees to the left. Place both of your fists to the right.

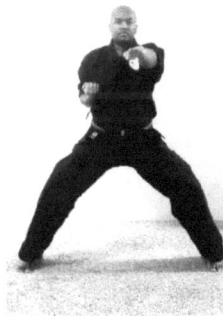

10. Chop with the left hand.

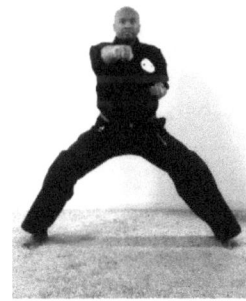

11. Punch with the right hand.

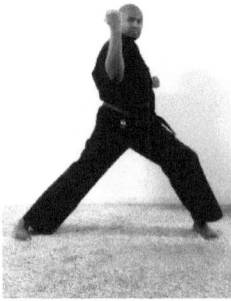

12. Shift into a front stance while turning 90 degrees to the left and performing an inside forearm block with the right hand.

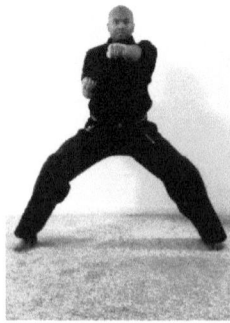

13. Shift into a horse stance while turning 90 degrees to the right and punching with the left hand.

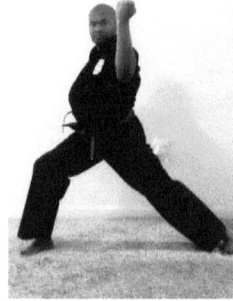

14. Shift into a front stance while turning 90 degrees to the right and performing an inside forearm block with the left hand.

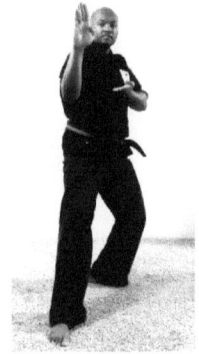

15. Perform a double knifehand block by taking a half step with the left foot in front of the right foot, then moving forward with the right foot into a back stance.

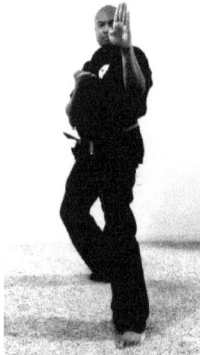

16. Step Forward
Back Stance
Double Knifehand Block

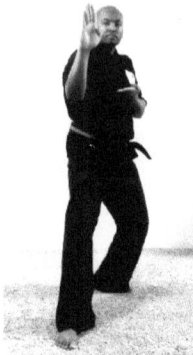

17. Step Forward
Back Stance
Double Knifehand Block

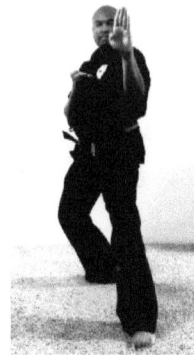

18. Step Back
Back Stance
Double Knifehand Block

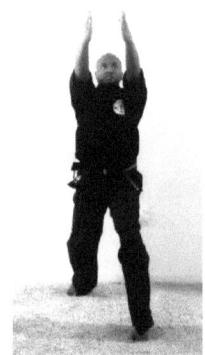

19. Shift forward into a front stance while keeping your left foot in front, and raise both of your open hands to the level of your neck.

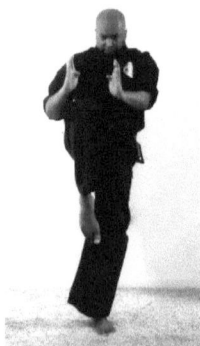

20. Strike with the right knee and pull both hands down beside the knee. Kihap!

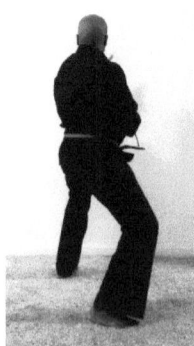

21. Turn Left 180 Degrees
Back Stance
Double Knifehand Block

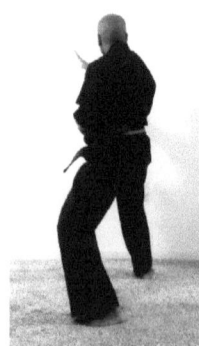

22. Step Forward
Back Stance
Double Knifehand Block

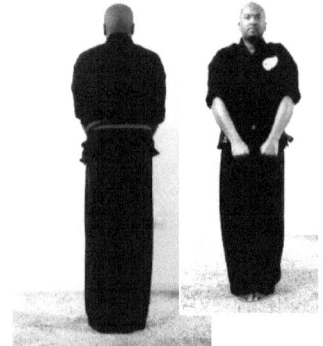

23. Lower both fists in front of you and pull the right foot back until both feet are together.

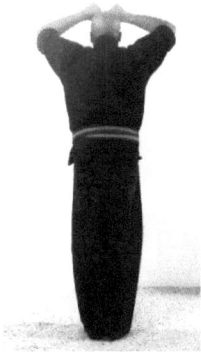

24. Raise both fists above your head.

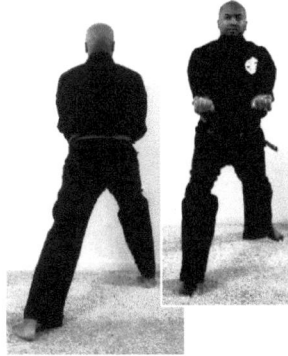

25. Perform a double punch by stepping into a front stance with your right foot.

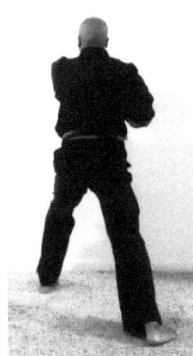

26. Step Forward Front Stance Middle Punch

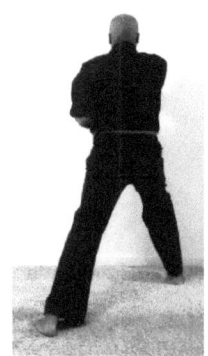

27. Step Forward Front Stance Middle Punch

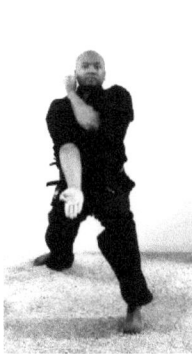

28. Turn left 180 degrees into a front stance and perform a low spear hand with your right hand while bringing your left hand beside your right ear.

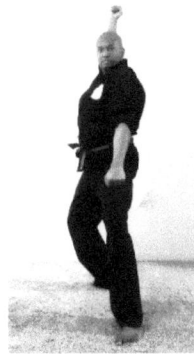

29. Shift into a back stance and pull your right arm behind you into an inside block while performing a low block with the left arm. *A*

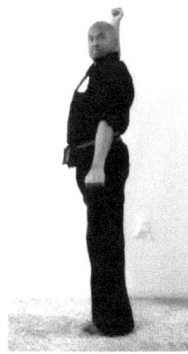

Bring your feet together by bringing your left foot to the side of your right foot. *B*

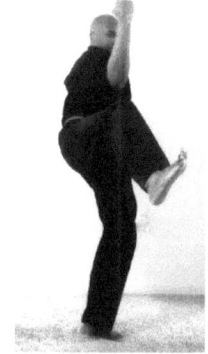

30. Turn 180 degrees to the left and perform an inside crescent kick with your right foot. *A*

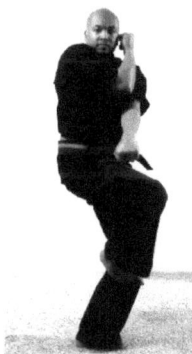

Cross both arms in front of your body, face the front, and balance on the left leg. *B*

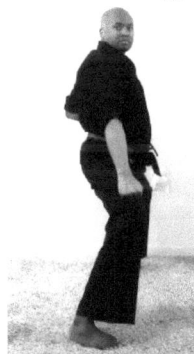

31. As you fall into a horse stance with your right foot, perform a low block with your right arm.

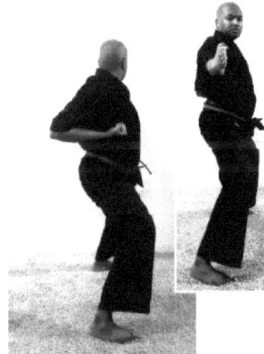

32. Turn 180 degrees to the left. Horse stance: extended left arm, open hand.

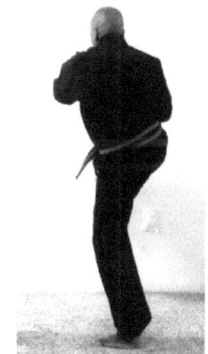

33. Turn 180 degrees to the left and perform an inside crescent kick with your right foot.

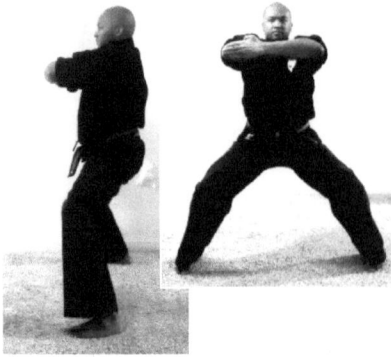

34. Strike your left open palm with your right elbow as you stamp down into a horse stance with the right foot.

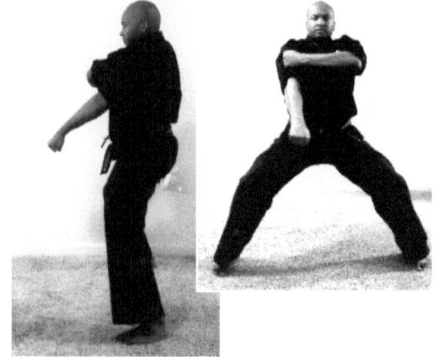

35. Low block with your right arm while remaining in a horse stance, keeping your left arm stationary.

A

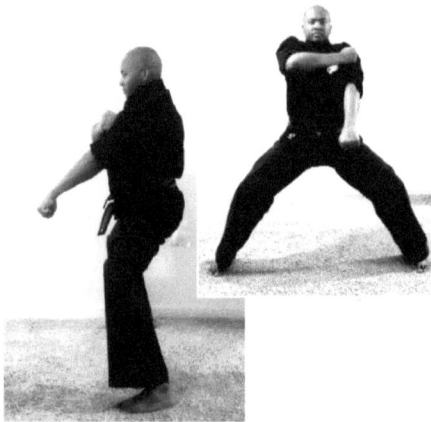

Switch your right arm with your left arm while remaining while in a horse stance.

B

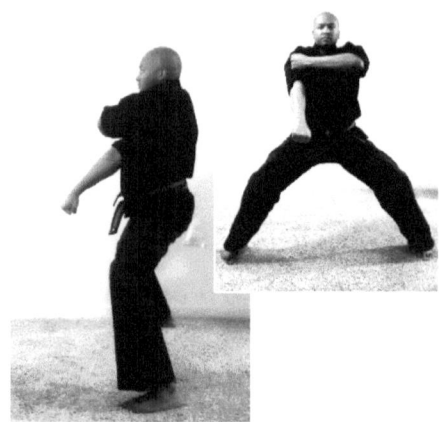

Switch your left arm with your right arm while remaining while in a horse stance.

C

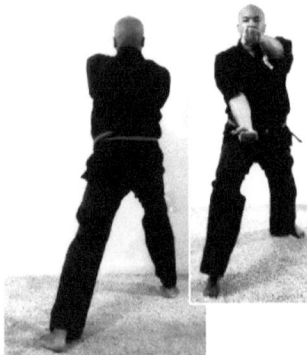

36. As you turn 90 degrees to the right and assume a front stance with your right foot out in front, execute a U-punch with the left arm on top and the right arm on bottom.

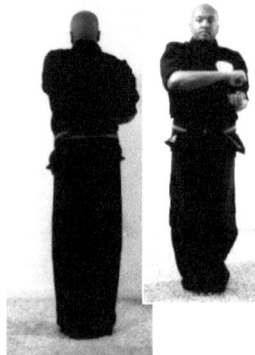

37. Bring your right foot to the side of your left foot and both of your fists to the right.

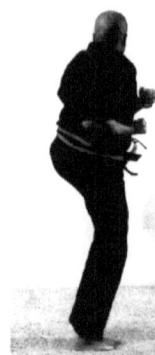

38. Perform an inside crescent kick with your left foot.

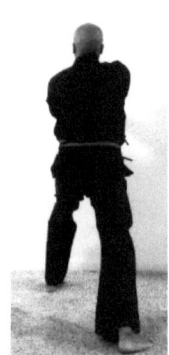

39. Step forward into a front stance with your left foot out in front, and execute a U-punch with the right arm on top and the left arm on bottom.

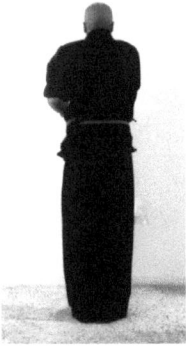

40. Bring your left foot to the side of your right foot and both of your fists to the left.

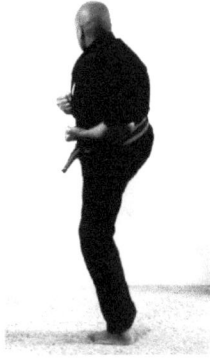

41. Perform an inside crescent kick with your right foot.

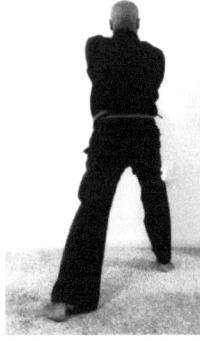

42. Step forward into a front stance with your right foot out in front, and execute a U-punch with the left arm on top and the right arm on bottom.

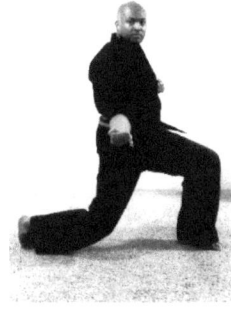

43. Perform a low backfist with your right hand while facing forward and 270 degrees to the left into a low front stance.

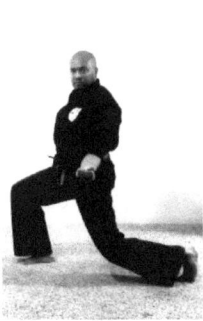

44. Perform a low backfist with your left hand while facing forward and 180 degrees to the right into a low front stance.

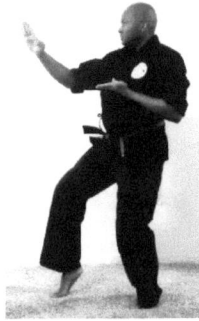

45. In a back stance, make a 90-degree turn to the right, and perform a double knifehand block.

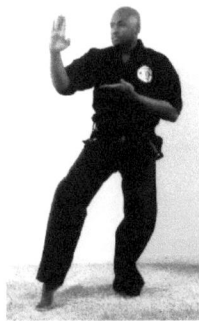

46. In a back stance, make a 45-degree turn to the right, step forward with your right foot, and double knifehand block.

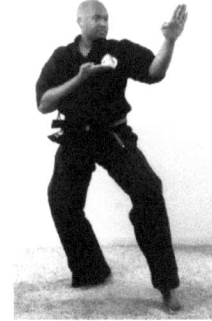

47. In a back stance, make a 45-degree turn to the left, step forward with your left foot, and double knifehand block. Kihap!

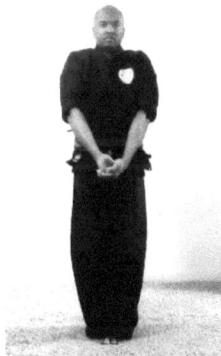

Finish: Ready Stance
(Bassai)

Resource

If you would like more information about the Black Karate Federation, please check out the website: **www.bkfwarriors.org**